Thyroid

EYE

Disease

Understanding Graves'

Ophthalmopathy

Elaine A. Moore

Printed in Victoria, Canada

First published in Canada in 2003 by
Your Health Press™, a division of Sarahealth.com Inc.
In association with Trafford Publishing.

Cover and text design: P. Krulicki, Colborne Communications

IMPORTANT NOTICE:
The purpose of this book is to educate. It is sold with the understanding that the author and publisher shall have neither liability nor responsibility for any injury caused or alleged to be caused directly or indirectly by the information contained in this book. While every effort has been made to ensure its accuracy, the book's contents should not be construed as medical advice. Each person's health needs are unique. To obtain recommendations appropriate to your particular situation, please consult a qualified health care provider. The herbal remedies recommended in this book are for education purposes only and should not be used without consulting a qualified expert in herbal medicine.

National Library of Canada Cataloguing in Publication

Moore, Elaine A., 1948-
        Thyroid eye disease : understanding Graves'
ophthalmopathy / Elaine A. Moore.

Includes bibliographical references and index.
ISBN 1-4120-0911-1

        1. Thyroid eye disease.   I. Title.

RE715.T48M66 2003   617.7   C2003-904794-6

This book was published *on-demand* in cooperation with Trafford Publishing.
On-demand publishing is a unique process and service of making a book available for retail sale to the public taking advantage of on-demand manufacturing and Internet marketing. **On-demand publishing** includes promotions, retail sales, manufacturing, order fulfilment, accounting and collecting royalties on behalf of the author.

Suite 6E, 2333 Government St., Victoria, B.C. V8T 4P4, CANADA

Phone	250-383-6864	Toll-free	1-888-232-4444 (Canada & US)
Fax	250-383-6804	E-mail	sales@trafford.com
Web site	www.trafford.com	TRAFFORD PUBLISHING IS A DIVISION OF TRAFFORD HOLDINGS LTD.
Trafford Catalogue #03-1280		www.trafford.com/robots/03-1280.html

10   9   8   7   6   5   4

OTHER BOOKS BY ELAINE A. MOORE

Graves' Disease, A Practical Guide, with Lisa M. Moore, McFarland & Company (2001)

Autoimmune Diseases & Their Environmental Triggers, McFarland & Company (2002)

Encyclopedia of Alzheimer's Disease, with Lisa M. Moore, McFarland & Company (2002)

OTHER YOUR HEALTH PRESS™ TITLES

Stopping Cancer at the Source by M. Sara Rosenthal, Ph.D. (2001)
Women and Unwanted Hair by M. Sara Rosenthal, Ph.D. (2001)
Living Well with Celiac Disease: Abundance Beyond Wheat and Gluten by Claudine Crangle (2002)
The Thyroid Cancer Book by M. Sara Rosenthal, Ph.D. (2002)
Living Well with an Ostomy by Elizabeth Rayson (2003)

Soon to be released...

Pediatric Glaucoma and Cataract Disease: Your Questions Answered by The Pediatric Glaucoma and Cataract Disease Foundation and edited by Alex Levin, M.D., F.R.C.P., Director, Ophthalmology, The Hospital for Sick Children (2003)
Healing Injuries the Natural Way: How to Mend Bones, Muscles, Tendons and More by Michelle Cook (2003)
Menopause Before 40: Coping with Premature Ovarian Failure by Karin Banerd (2003)

ABOUT THE AUTHOR

Elaine Moore is a Medical Technologist, MT (ASCP), with more than 30 years experience working in hospital laboratories. The mother of two grown children, Elaine, her husband Rick, and their three boxers live in the mountains of Colorado.

DEDICATION

This book is dedicated to all those who suffer from thyroid related eye disorders or who are in some way affected by their consequences.

TABLE OF CONTENTS

Acknowledgements 9

Introduction..11

Chapter 1: What is Graves' Ophthalmopathy? 15

Chapter 2: Subtypes of GO 27

Chapter 3: Signs and Symptoms 31

Chapter 4: Classifying GO..43

Chapter 5: Orbital Anatomy & Inflammatory Orbital Disease.........49

Chapter 6: Cellular & Immune System Changes 63

Chapter 7: The Autoimmune Element 67

Chapter 8: Risk Factors..75

Chapter 9: Diagnosis 83

Chapter 10: Conventional Treatment Options 101

Chapter 11: Complementary Therapy in GO 129

Chapter 12: Psychosocial Factors: the Survivors 139

Resources 157

Glossary 163

Bibliography...175

Index 179

ACKNOWLEDGEMENTS

I'd like to take this opportunity to thank my publisher M. Sara Rosenthal of Your Health Press™ for bringing the need for a book on thyroid related eye disorders to my attention. I'd also like to thank Mary Shomon for suggesting that I write it. I'm also indebted to the Eye Institute of the National Institutes of Health for generously sharing their resources. And I'd like to thank all of the many patients with Graves' Ophthalmopathy (GO), especially Jody, Mary, Mona, Bill, Laura and my other friends who kindly shared their personal experiences dealing with GO. And special thanks go to Dr. Charles Soparkar for graciously reviewing the chapter on conventional treatment.

I'd also like to extend hearty thanks to the many thyroid patients who have approached me with questions and concerns. These questions and concerns shaped the contents of this book. And, I'd like to thank my talented friend, the clinical chemist Marvin G. Miller, for illustrating *Thyroid Eye Disease*. His pictures portray more than words ever could. Last but in no way least, I can't forget to thank my family, especially my husband, for understanding the pressure of deadlines and for understanding my need to teach others about the nature of autoimmune disease, including the important role that education and self-care play in the healing process.

INTRODUCTION

*T*hyroid *Eye Disease:Understanding Graves Ophthalmopathy* is intended as an educational resource and guide for patients with Graves' ophthalmopathy (GO), an inflammatory eye disorder that often precedes, accompanies, or follows autoimmune thyroid disease. Although the thyroid and eye conditions usually occur simultaneously, GO may occur as much as ten years before and 20 years after the initial thyroid disorder emerges.

The most common types of thyroid disease occur when the thyroid gland fails to secrete adequate thyroid hormone, causing a condition known as hypothyroidism; alternately, the thyroid gland may secrete excess thyroid hormone, causing a condition known as hyperthyroidism. Graves' disease is an autoimmune hyperthyroid disorder and the most common cause of hyperthyroidism.

GO primarily occurs in patients with Graves' disease (80 percent of all cases); and in a smaller number of individuals with Hashimoto's thyroiditis (HT), an autoimmune hypothyroid disorder. GO may also occur in people who have no signs of thyroid disease (these people are said to have euthyroid Graves' disease). Approximately ten percent of all GO occurs in people with euthyroid Graves' disease, and another ten percent occurs in people with HT.

Thyroid associated eye disorders are known by a number of different names, including Graves' ophthalmopathy (GO); thyroid eye disease (TED); thyroid associated ophthalmopathy (TAO); dysthyroid orbitopathy; thyroid ophthalmopathy; immune exophthalmos; and Graves' eye disease. In this book, the condition of thyroid related eye disease will be referred to simply as GO.

Both autoimmune thyroid disease (AITD) and GO, like most autoimmune disorders, result from a combination of genetic and environmental factors. That is, individuals with a certain combination of genes develop AITD and GO when they're exposed to certain environmental triggers, including stress, infectious agents, iodine, interferon and interleukin medications and sex steroids. Thyroid autoantibodies that contribute to the development of AITD also play a significant role in the development of GO, particularly the congestive form of GO. A complex disease, which is unique in each individual, GO may affect the eyelids, the orbital muscles, the orbital connective tissue and the orbital fat deposits.

My goal in writing *Thyroid Eye Disease: Understanding Graves Ophthamopathy* is to educate, support and empower patients with GO. Intended as an overall guide, this book describes all facets of GO—including the development, signs, symptoms, diagnostic tests, risk factors, conventional and complementary treatment options, complications, and psychosocial manifestations of GO.

Chapter 1 describes what it means to have Graves' ophthalmopathy thyroid related eye disease and introduces the reader to a list of associated medical words and terms. Chapter 2 explains the two primary subtypes of GO and their differences. Chapter 3 looks at the signs and symptoms associated with GO. Chapter 4 describes how GO is classified and the usefulness of these stages. Chapter 5 describes how the eye's tissues and cells work together to create vision, and it describes the changes seen in inflammatory GO. Chapter 6 describes the immune system and its cells and explains how immune system changes contribute to GO. Chapter 7 describes the autoimmune process that results in the congestive, inflammatory form of GO. Chapter 8 describes the genetic, environmental and lifestyle factors that contribute to GO development. Chapter 9 describes the clinical picture, laboratory and imaging tests used to help diagnosis in GO. Chapter 10 describes conventional treatment options and explains their use in the various disease stages. Chapter 11 describes the use of complementary medicine in GO. And chapter 12 describes the psychosocial effects of living with GO. Also included are patient anecdotes, illustrations, a resource section, glossary and index.

In any disease state, but particularly in diseases with an autoimmune origin, knowledge is empowering. Armed with an understanding of the endocrine, environmental, genetic and immunological factors that lead to GO, you can better understand how this disease develops and realize the importance of your own role in the healing process.

Studies show that the amount of time and energy you invest in your own healing directly affects your outcome. With several therapeutic options available for GO, you must be able to weigh benefits against side effects and have an active voice in your own treatment plans. Recent advances in immunology have demonstrated that the endocrine, immune and nervous systems work in harmony, and anything that influences one system influences the others. Thus, the role of dietary changes, supplements, and the avoidance of environmental triggers must all be taken into consideration. By learning what foods promote inflammation or how chronic stress harms the immune system, you'll soon be able to modulate your body's own immune responses.

While usually mild and manageable, the signs and symptoms of GO are often more debilitating than their related thyroid disorders. Furthermore, thyroid related eye disorders have other ramifications besides the obvious medical concerns. The resulting cosmetic disfigurement can cause psychosocial distress, inability to work and considerable financial hardship during the active disease stages. Even after the disease has stabilized and resolved, one or more corrective surgeries may be required.

While various treatments are available to treat GO, the period in which their use is beneficial and the order in which treatments should be administered are as important as the therapy itself. This book includes a thorough description of treatment options—be they conventional or complementary—with an added emphasis on the role of self-care.

While the intricate workings of the immune system are complex and beyond the scope of this book, several sections, particularly in chapters 6 and 7, describe how the immune system contributes to GO development. Other sections, especially in chapters 8 and 11, show how diet, stress and other environmental factors influence immune system health. Adopting a lifestyle that promotes immune system health is the first step when it comes to healing and remission in GO.

While the disease process in GO is indeed complex and appears mysterious at first glance, the steps that lead to GO are logical and orderly. More importantly, the effects of GO and the severity of its symptoms are partially under your control. Some of the most powerful healing tools, such as avoiding sugar to prevent inflammation or drinking sufficient water to prevent dryness and tearing, are easy. Maintaining appropriate thyroid hormone levels will also affect your disease course. Avoiding cigarette smoke may be more difficult, but the results can be particularly dramatic. Incorporating helpful lifestyle changes and modulating the immune system are achievable goals. Let this book be your guide to both understanding how GO develops and learning how you can influence its course and attain both remission and recovery.

1
WHAT ARE THYROID ASSOCIATED EYE DISEASE AND GRAVES' OPHTHALMOPATHY?

Shortly after Jody, a political activist in her forties, had radioiodine I131 ablative treatment for hyperthyroidism related to Graves' disease (autoimmune hyperthyroidism), she learned that this particular treatment was linked to the development of Graves' ophthalmopathy (GO). As the months went by and she struggled to control her symptoms of radioiodine-induced hypothyroidism, she assumed that she was no longer at risk for developing thyroid related eye disease.

Although Jody complained to her support group friends about depression, which had been triggered by her severe hypothyroidism, Jody told her friends that she was fortunate that at least she'd never developed GO. Unfortunately, however, during her sixth post-ablative year, her eyes began to tear frequently and she noticed a feeling of grittiness and occasional pain in her eyeball (ocular pain). She was astonished when her endocrinologist remarked that her eye symptoms were likely related to her thyroid condition.

When she consulted an ophthalmologist (a doctor who specializes in diagnosing and treating eye diseases), she learned that she was experiencing early symptoms of GO. That's when Jody began a crash course, learning everything she could about her condition. In chapter 12, you'll learn more about Jody and her success using a non-traditional treatment approach for her GO.

In Chapter 1, you'll learn, as Jody did, what it means to have the thyroid related eye disease commonly known as Graves' ophthalmopathy (GO). In addition this chapter defines some of the terms frequently used in discussing the symptoms and circumstances surrounding GO.

Graves' Ophthalmopathy

Graves' ophthalmopathy is an inflammatory ocular disorder with a wide range of symptoms. The most common symptoms include staring, proptosis, dryness, grittiness, and eyelid retraction. GO may affect the extraocular muscles and connective tissue that support the eye; the blood vessels and nerves that serve the eye; and the eyelids that protect the eye.

In GO, inflammation or congestion typically affects the connective tissues, fat deposits, and the muscles of the eye. These components are situated in the parabulbar (on the sides of the eyeball) and retrobulbar (behind the eyeball) areas. Inflammation occurs when immune system cells cluster and aggregate in these sites of orbital tissue. It is widely accepted that GO is an autoimmune disorder that runs its own independent course, which may run parallel to the thyroid disorder. This is supported by the cellular or immune system changes seen in eye (orbital) tissue in patients with GO.

The Mechanism in GO

In GO, one or more of the six ocular muscles that move the eye become enlarged. These muscles normally cannot be seen on the surface. They originate behind the eye at the peak of the eye socket and attach to the eye just behind the cornea. A thin layer of tissue known as the conjunctiva covers the eye muscles. The muscles may become visible as the blood vessels over their anterior (front) portion become prominent due to the muscle enlargement.

The fatty tissue present in the eye also enlarges in GO as it becomes filled with fluid and white blood cells. The increased volume of both the eye muscles and orbital fat leads to increased retrobulbar pressure within the bony orbital cage or socket that surrounds the eye. Consequently, the eye's tissues become inflamed, reddened and swollen. The crowded orbital cavity displaces the eyeball, pushing it forward. This causes a bulging of the eye known as exophthalmos or proptosis. The enlarged muscles and additional fluids restrict muscle movement. Usually, one muscle is frozen into a fixed position while the other muscles are able to move freely. This impaired muscle motility interferes with muscle alignment and causes diplopia (double vision). Usually, in the diplopia related to GO, one image is seen on top of the other.

With muscle enlargement, the globe or eyeball is also pushed forward, causing a characteristic "stare." The muscles may also stiffen, causing the eyelids to retract or pull away from the colored portion of the eye. Blood vessels can also become prominent and contribute to redness. The enlarged muscles may also press on the optic nerve and interfere with vision. And in extreme cases, optic nerve dysfunction (optic neuropathy) may occur.

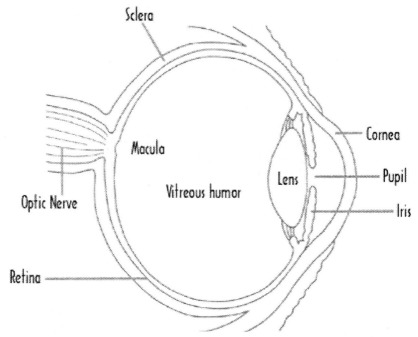

Diagram of the Eye. Copyright © National Eye Institute, National Institutes of Health. Reprinted with permission.

How GO Develops

As the muscles enlarge, three distinct events can occur: 1) the eyeball gets pushed forward, causing a prominent stare or proptosis; 2) the muscles may become stiff with impaired motility causing eye motility problems, including diplopia; and 3) the muscles may press on the optic nerve and interfere with vision. One or more of these possible events occurs in patients with GO.

Inflammation

Inflammation is a process characterized by congestion or swelling initi-ated by the immune system. In the inflammatory response, white blood cells cluster at the point of injury or at the site of specific antigens (in GO, the specific antigen is TSH protein found on orbital cells). In the process of inflammation, immune system cells release immune system chemicals called cytokines. Cytokines contribute to swelling and fluid retention (edema), and they prolong the inflammatory process.

A Unique Disorder

No two people with GO follow the same disease course. Most researchers agree that thyroid associated eye disorders are self-limiting. This means the active inflammatory process in GO eventually resolves although it may leave a number of cosmetic changes that ultimately require corrective surgery.

Symptoms in GO can be of variable severity, causing several mild to severe flare-ups during a short disease course. Alternately, symptoms can persist incessantly, diligently moving through progressive phases and lasting up to five years before stabilizing. Another unusual facet of GO is the body's own attempt to heal orbital congestion by "spontaneously decompressing"—causing the eye to bulge forward in an effort to make more room in the orbital cavity. The result is exophthalmos or proptosis.

Writing in *Endocrine Emergencies*, Dr. R. Patrick Yeatts explains that, "Often the patient who is unable to "decompress" spontaneously (i.e., the patient with minimal proptosis) displays the most profound visual loss. An increased resistance to displacement of the globe can be observed clinically. In such a patient, the forward movement of the globe is limited by the extraocular muscles, and additional decompression limited by a taut orbital septum."

Thus, appearances in GO can be deceiving. Patients with the least significant cosmetic changes may experience the most serious complications. Therefore, it is essential that patients with symptoms of ocular pain, blurred vision or loss of color vision contact their physicians immediately so that they can be examined and receive prompt treatment if it is indicated.

The Name Game

While the technical name for thyroid related eye disorders is Graves' ophthalmopathy or GO, this condition is referred to by many other names. Other names used to describe GO include: dysthyroid ophthalmopathy; endocrine ophthalmopathy; dysthyroid orbitopathy; thyroid ophthalmopathy; orbital ophthalmopathy; thyroid associated ophthalmopathy

(TAO); thyroid eye disease (TED); and Graves' eye disease. When GO occurs in patients who show no evidence or past history of thyroid dysfunction, the disorder is known as euthyroid Graves' disease.

Who Develops GO?

Estimates of how many people have GO vary depending on several factors. Most important is the sensitivity of the detection method. When patients with Graves' disease are examined for signs of GO using sensitive imaging techniques, such as computed tomography (CT), magnetic resonance imaging (MRI) or ultrasonography, nearly all of them show signs of extraocular muscle involvement.

Despite the frequency of these signs, many of these patients have no clinical symptoms. Overall, less than half of Graves' disease patients end up developing clinically significant GO. Only about 35 percent of Graves' disease patients and only about 2 percent of patients with Hashimoto's thyroiditis go on to develop clinically significant GO. And of those who do develop clinically significant GO, only about 3 to 5 percent go on to develop severe eye disease.

If eyelid signs, such as lid retraction, are excluded, 10 to 25 percent of Graves' patients show clinically significant eye disease. When eyelid signs are included, 30 to 45 percent of Graves' disease patients develop clinically significant eye disease.

The incidence of GO was determined for residents of Olmsted County, Minnesota for the years 1976 through 1990. A total of 120 cases were found with 16 cases occurring in women and 2.9 cases occurring in men for each 100,000 persons. In women, peak incidence occurred in the age groups 40 to 44 years and 60 to 64 years. In men, peak incidence occurred in the age groups 45 to 49 years and 65 to 69 years. No seasonal variation was noted

Linking GO with Thyroid Disease

Of all clinically significant cases of GO, 80 percent occur in patients with Graves' disease, 10 percent occur in patients with Hashimoto's thyroiditis (an autoimmune hypothyroid disorder), and 10 percent occur in patients with no signs of thyroid disease. While approximately 25 percent of patients with Graves' disease will develop GO; approximately 2 percent of patients with Hashimoto's thyroiditis develop this order.

Thyroid Eye Disease

On rare occasions, patients with primary hypothyroidism, thyroid cancer, and patients with other forms of thyroiditis may have eye findings consistent with GO. Although women are much more likely to develop GO, men are more likely to have severe eye disease. Thyroid related eye disorders are also more likely to occur in cigarette smokers. Studies also show that smokers are more likely to have a relapse from Graves' disease after treatment, and their course of GO is typically worse than that of non-smokers. In addition, studies show that an individual's thyroid antibodies and immune system genes play a major role in determining whether they will develop GO and, if they do, how severe their symptoms will be.

Patients of any age may develop GO, although children tend to have milder forms of GO than adults. In one Swiss study of 196 Graves' disease patients, the average age of patients who did not go on to develop GO was 41.9 years. The average age of patients who developed GO was 41.6 years.

Euthyroid Graves' Disease

Conversely, in about ten percent of cases, GO has been known to develop years before the thyroid disorder emerges. This condition is known as euthyroid Graves' disease. In euthyroid Graves' disease, patients show no signs of having a thyroid disorder although nearly all of these patients will show evidence of thyroid autoimmunity if they are tested for the complete spectrum of thyroid antibodies (thyroid peroxidase antibodies; thyroglobulin antibodies; blocking, stimulating and binding TSH receptor antibodies; and thyroid growth immunoglobulins). Thyroid antibodies are described further in chapter 6.

Upon close investigation, some thyrotoxic patients who appear to have no signs of thyroid overactivity may actually have Hashitoxicosis. Hashitoxicosis is a self-limited form of thyrotoxicosis in which the inflammatory changes in the thyroid cause the release of stored thyroid hormone. Since the gland is not hyperfunctioning, most patients become hypothyroid after the stored thyroid hormones are used up.

The Timeframe

Most patients develop GO within 18 months of their initial diagnosis of thyroid disease, with most of these patients developing GO during the same year that they developed thyroid disease. However, GO can develop as much as twenty years later, especially in patients who have had radioiodine ablation treatment for hyperthyroidism. Symptoms of GO may develop at any time in patients with Hashimoto's thyroiditis. In these patients, severe GO is most likely to occur in patients who are under-treated and remain hypothyroid, or who have high titers of TSH receptor antibodies.

GO Terminology

Besides having many aliases, Graves' ophthalmopathy has its own peculiar vocabulary. While many of the terms related to GO are defined in the glossary as well as in the relevant chapters, the following section includes definitions for a number of conditions that may be associated with GO. This compilation is intended to help describe GO and to familiarize you with these terms when you encounter them in later chapters and to help you in understanding copies of your medical records.

Bilateral Symmetry

Bilateral is a term meaning that both eyes are affected. Symmetric or symmetrical denotes that both eyes are equally affected. Thyroid eye disease is the most common cause of bilateral, symmetric proptosis (eyeball bulging) in adults. However, not all incidences of bilateral proptosis are caused by GO, and not all incidences of proptosis in GO are bilateral or symmetrical. Most patients with GO present with asymmetrical eye disease, meaning that one eye is affected more than the other.

Blurred Vision

Visual blurring is considered a serious symptom when it occurs in GO. It may occur as a result of alterations to the tear film, irritation of the cornea, or muscle imbalances not related to diplopia. Visual blurring can also be a sign of optic neuropathy, which is a potential complication of GO.

Congestive Infiltration

Congestive infiltration refers to the subtype of GO related to immune system changes. Congestive infiltrative disease is more serious than the more common subtype of GO, which is caused by thyroid hormone imbalances, especially excess thyroid hormone. In congestive GO, deposits of immune system chemicals and immune system cells infiltrate orbital tissue, causing inflammation. This results in an increased orbital volume and increased ocular pressure.

Thyroid Eye Disease

Diplopia

Diplopia is a condition of seeing double (double vision), and results from extraocular muscle changes that cause overlapping fields of vision. Diplopia may also occur after ocular surgery due to changes in muscle alignment. Double vision is usually due to misalignment of the eyes. Most people with GO experience a condition known as binocular diplopia. Binocular diplopia can be corrected when either eye is covered. Monocular diplopia (diplopia that persists when viewing with one eye) is unusual, and is most often caused by an abnormality in the cornea or lens, and rarely by a detached retina.

Euthyroid

Euthyroid refers to a condition characterized by normal thyroid function tests (normal levels of FT4, T3 or FT3, and TSH). Patients with active thyroid disease become euthyroid when their thyroid levels are kept under control with treatment, including thyroid replacement hormone or anti-thyroid drugs. However, because TSH may take many weeks to rise after their thyrotoxicosis is corrected, patients on anti-thyroid drug therapy for hyperthyroidism are considered euthyroid when their FT4 and T3 or FT3 levels fall within the normal or reference range. When GO occurs in individuals who are euthyroid and have no symptoms or past history of thyroid disease, they are said to have euthyroid Graves' disease.

Exophthalmos

(See Proptosis.)

External Beam Radiotherapy

External beam radiotherapy (XRT) is a form of therapy commonly used to treat symptoms of congestive GO. In this form of therapy, patients are treated with external radiation over a period of time—usually ten weeks. External beam radiotherapy selectively destroys the lymphocytes that are present in orbital tissue and responsible for inflammation. External beam radiotherapy is only effective when used during the active disease state when lymphocytes are actively infiltrating orbital tissue.

Extraocular Muscle

The six ocular muscles that support the globe of the eye are commonly referred to as extraocular muscles because they originate away from the globe and exist as separate structures. The extraocular muscles include the levator palpebrae superioris (levator), rectus superior, rectus inferior, rectus medialis, rectus lateralis, and obliquus superior (oblique) muscles. The extraocular muscles become enlarged in congestive GO. This change initiates the disease process in GO.

Eyelid Retraction

In eyelid retraction, the eyelids tend to pull back or away from the eye. Eyelid retraction may be directly related to hyperthyroidism. In this case, excess thyroid hormone causes sympathetic nerve stimulation, which causes the eyelids to retract. When this happens, unless scarring occurs, eyelid retraction resolves when the thyroid hormone levels are corrected. Alternately, eyelid retraction may result from direct muscle involvement (impaired muscle motility) related to inflammation. Upper lid elevation, particularly when looking down, is very characteristic of GO.

Graves' Disease

Graves' disease is an autoimmune hyperthyroid disorder that may also affect the eyes, skin and muscular system. Graves' disease is caused by thyroid autoantibodies that stimulate the TSH receptor, bypassing the normal mechanisms that regulate thyroid hormone and causing thyroid cells to produce and secrete excess thyroid hormone. The same stimulating TSH receptor antibodies that cause Graves' hyperthyroidism cause GO as well as a skin condition known as pretibial myxedema.

Hashimoto's Thyroiditis

Hashimoto's thyroiditis (HT) is an autoimmune hypothyroid disorder caused by an inflammatory process that destroys thyroid cells and interferes with their normal functions. Ten percent of all cases of GO occur in patients with HT.

Optic Neuropathy

The optic nerve connects the eye to the brain producing images of vision. Optic neuropathy refers to inflammation or damage to the optic nerve, resulting in compression and vision loss. Optic neuropathy is one of the more serious complications of GO because it can interfere with vision and lead to blindness. Symptoms of optic neuropathy include blurred vision, decreased color vision, and decreased visual acuity, which is characterized by the appearance of holes or shadows in the field of vision.

An inability to distinguish the color red is one of the first signs of color vision loss. This is characterized by color desaturation, a condition in which red tones appear pink or "washed out." Researchers note that the ocular fundus in optic neuropathy is usually normal, although disc edema, choroidal folds, and optic disc pallor may be seen.

Orbital Decompression

Decompression is a term that basically means "relief from compression." In GO, chemical and cellular deposits create pressure in the orbital cavity. To accommodate this, the eye cavity undergoes attempts to spontaneously decompress by moving the eye forward in its socket causing proptosis. In orbital decompression surgery, the orbital cavity is surgically expanded to accommodate the increase in orbital tissue and relieve proptosis. Orbital decompression involves the removal of the orbital bones. This allows the orbital tissue to expand into surrounding spaces previously occupied by bone, such as the lateral wall or roof, or by the ethmoid and maxillary sinuses.

Periorbital Edema

Edema (fluid retention) is characterized by swelling. In periorbital edema, any of the tissue surrounding the eye may be affected. Edema in GO results from enlargement of ocular muscles and impaired venous circulation. Periorbital edema also occurs in hypothyroidism-related GO.

Proptosis

Proptosis, a condition resulting from anterior or forward displacement of the globes of one or both eyes, causing abnormal protrusion, is also referred to as exophthalmos. Proptosis occurs as the orbital cavity spontaneously decompresses in an attempt to house the extra accumulations of tissue and fluid that occur in congestive GO.

The degree of proptosis depends on how much soft tissue (both extraocular muscle and connective tissue) fills the orbital cavity. Proptosis also occurs when deposits of orbital fat, a chemical known as glycosaminoglycan (GAG), and white blood cells infiltrate orbital tissue, expanding tissue volume. An increase in orbital volume as small as 4 ml can cause as much as 6 mm of proptosis. Proptosis greater than 21 mm as measured by the Hertel Exophthalmometer is considered abnormal.

Strabismus

Strabismus is an ophthalmic condition characterized by an inability of the eyes to focus together because of an imbalance in the muscles that control eye movement. Strabismus, which typically causes squinting, may affect one or both eyes.

Horizontal strabismus occurs when the eyes are unable to move together laterally, causing a condition of cross-eye if the eye turns inward and walleye if the eye turns outward. Vertical strabismus occurs when the eye rolls upward or downward in it socket. In torsional strabismus the eyes are unable to rotate together about their optical axes. In patients with GO, strabismus may ultimately lead to diplopia.

Radioiodine Ablation

Radioiodine ablation refers to a specific treatment for hyperthyroidism or thyroid cancer in which radioactive iodine (radioisotope of iodine), usually I-131, is used to ablate or destroy thyroid cells, effectively reducing the amount of thyroid tissue available to produce thyroid hormone. Radioiodine ablation may increase the risk of developing GO because it releases components of the thyroid gland into the bloodstream, including stimulating TSH receptor antibodies. TSH receptor antibodies induce the development of congestive GO. This is most likely to happen in the small group of patients with significant GO prior to radioiodine treatment.

Thyroiditis

Thyroiditis refers to inflammation of the thyroid gland. Thyroiditis is related to both hyperthyroidism and hypothyroidism. Thyroiditis may result from autoimmune processes or it may be caused by bacterial or viral infections. Bacterial and viral thyroiditis are generally not associated with GO, although symptoms related to abnormal thyroid hormone levels may occur.

During the postpartum period, from five to ten percent of all women develop a transient postpartum thyroiditis (PPT) that can be accompanied by symptoms of GO. PPT, which generally resolves within one year, is thought to be autoimmune in nature and is related to immune system changes that occur during pregnancy. PPT can cause symptoms of hypothyroidism or hyperthyroidism, or sometimes hyperthyroidism followed by hypothyroidism, before eventually resolving.

Thyrotoxicosis

Thyrotoxicosis is a clinical syndrome caused by excess levels of thyroid hormone in the blood. Thyrotoxicosis may cause symptoms in all of the body's organs. General symptoms of thyrotoxicosis include weight loss, fatigue, heat intolerance, irritability, palpitations, tachycardia, atrial fibrillation, tremor, agitation, loss of libido, menstrual changes, nausea, eye changes, and hair, nail and skin changes. Hyperthyroidism refers to overactivity of the thyroid gland as one cause of thyrotoxicosis; however, thyrotoxicosis can occur without hyperthyroidism, such as when taking excessive dosages of thyroid hormone pills, or during hashitoxicosis.

2
SUBTYPES OF GO

There are two distinct subtypes of GO. The first is related to stimulation of the sympathetic nervous system caused by abnormal thyroid hormone levels; and the second, a more serious congestive or infiltrative type of eye disease caused by immune system changes. In the milder variations of the disease, which are primarily related to high levels of thyroid hormone, symptoms generally resolve when the thyroid condition is treated and thyroid hormone levels are returned to the normal range.

In the more severe congestive, infiltrative disorder GO runs its own course, independent of the thyroid disorder. While generally progressing in discrete predictable stages, the course of the congestive eye disorder may vary considerably, merely causing mild periodic flare-ups. Because it is autoimmune in origin, the congestive form of GO can cause symptoms that wax and wane, growing worse in times of stress.

Although my own experiences with congestive GO were mild, my symptoms varied considerably. Some days I would wake up with badly swollen eyes, and on other days my eyes would merely look puffy. The light sensitivity or photobia that I've had since childhood, however, has never receded. I'm forced to wear dark sunglasses year round along with a perpetual frown (commonly known as a thyroid frown).

GO Related to Abnormal Thyroid Hormone Levels

The spastic disorder, which causes symptoms of dryness, tearing, staring, puffiness (periorbital edema), and twitching, generally resolves when thyroid hormone levels are corrected. Symptoms can occur when patients are hyperthyroid or hypothyroid, although in most cases this type of GO is related to excess thyroid hormone.

Hypothyroid patients are most likely to show symptoms of periorbital edema, which results in a swelling that can completely circle the eye and cause deep pouches beneath the lower lids. Hyperthyroid patients and also hypothyroid patients taking excess thyroid hormone generally develop a staring appearance and experience eyelid retraction.

Sympathetic Nervous System Effects

Patients with Graves' disease (autoimmune hyperthyroidism) frequently exhibit spastic symptoms when their thyroid hormone levels are elevated. Up to 90 percent of patients with active Graves' disease are reported to exhibit a prominent stare. The effects of excess thyroid hormone on the sympathetic nervous system are responsible. These effects are often referred to as catecholamine (epinephrine and norepinephrine) stimulation.

The resulting sympathetic overactivity causes contraction of the levator muscle of the eye, causing a fixed stare, which has been reported to respond well to drugs known as beta adrenergic blocking agents (beta blockers), such as propranolol.

Hypothyroidism

Hyperthyroid patients who become hypothyroid as a result of ablative treatment or from natural disease progression often exhibit symptoms of GO, particularly periorbital edema. These symptoms persist until thyroid hormone levels are returned to the normal range. Failure to maintain normal thyroid hormone levels during therapy for hyperthyroidism also contributes to the development of congestive GO.

Because thyroid hormone is necessary for all of the body's functions, including the movement of fluids through the body, thyroid hormone deficiency causes impaired venous and lymphatic circulation. Consequently, fluids are retained causing the skin to become puffy and swollen. The word myxedema, which is sometimes used to describe hypothyroidism, refers to the waterlogged appearance of the skin in hypothyroidism.

Euthyroid Patients

In patients who are euthyroid (normal thyroid hormone levels), stare may occur as a result of severe proptosis. Patients with a past incidence of hyperthyroidism that caused fibrosis and scarring of the levator muscles that raise the eyelids, may also exhibit this prominent stare.

Instances of GO that are caused by abnormal thyroid hormone levels represent slightly less than 20 percent of all cases of clinically significant GO. It is the congestive form of GO that follows its own course and causes the most serious complications. Some ophthalmologists only refer to the congestive forms of GO as true ophthalmopathy. Eye symptoms caused by thyroid hormone imbalance are generally managed by an endocrinologist.

Congestive Autoimmune Related GO

The congestive infiltrative disorder referred to in the previous section is caused by immune system changes that produce inflammation. In this form of GO, the immune system also causes cellular changes that ultimately cause the increased production of a sticky mucinous chemical substance known as glycosaminoglycan (GAG).

Deposits of GAG and white blood cells, particularly lymphocytes and macrophages, infiltrate the orbital area, lodging between tissue fibers and causing eye muscle enlargement. This results in an expansion of the orbital tissues that fill the bony orbital cavity that surrounds the eyeball. To accommodate this additional volume, most patients will experience a spontaneous decompression in which the eyeball pushes forward in an effort to relieve pressure.

This accommodation for space causes a bulging of the eye from its orbit known as proptosis. It also leads to congestion of the blood vessels supplying the orbital area, causing tearing, eye discomfort and blurred vision. If the orbital congestion and infiltration are severe enough, the orbital nerve may be compressed, causing diminished visual sharpness or acuity, loss of peripheral vision or visual field defects and reduced color vision.

Genetic differences and environmental triggers (including diet and stress), as well as different immunological profiles (the types of thyroid and, perhaps, other autoantibodies an individual has at the time), contribute to both the severity and course of GO. Consequently, all patients with GO have unique symptoms and a unique disease course.

GO Extras

"Extra" in this case is a medical prefix used to describe conditions or symptoms occurring away from their usual or ordinary source. For instance, Graves' ophthalmopathy is often referred to as an extrathyroidal symptom of Graves' disease because it occurs in an organ away from the thyroid gland. Extraocular muscle is a term commonly used to describe the eye muscles that are situated outside or away from the ocular orbit or eyeball. Situated behind the globe, these muscles support the eyeball and allow it to move.

The Disease Course

While symptoms related to thyroid hormone imbalance generally resolve when thyroid hormone levels are corrected, the congestive form of GO follows its own course independent of the eye disease. Some people may only experience occasional flare-ups although in most patients the disease is characterized by an active phase, a plateau phase and a recovery phase.

Symptoms of congestive disease are directly related to cellular and chemical changes caused by the immune system. The active phase of GO usually lasts for three to six months, although on rare occasions it can last as long as three years. The entire disease course of GO generally resolves within one to two years although it can persist for as long as five to ten years in rare instances.

A Self-Limiting Disorder

It is generally accepted that congestive GO is self-limiting, although the time frame for resolution varies. In one Swiss study of 196 Graves' disease patients, 81 patients developed GO. The mean observation period in which symptoms of GO occurred was 3.23 years, with a duration ranging from 1 up to 8.9 years. GO developed within 12 months of the hyperthyroid disorder in 70 percent of these patients. Of the 81 patients with GO, 53 received no therapy. Of these, 25 patients improved spontaneously, 26 showed no changes and 2 had symptoms of progressive deterioration.

In this study, only the patients with more severe forms of GO were administered treatment. Eleven of the original 81 patients were administered corticosteroids; of these, 7 improved, 3 did not change, and 1 patient worsened. Five of the 81 patients received orbital radiotherapy. Of these, 3 improved, and 2 showed no changes.

This study supported the findings of other studies showing that most patients with GO experience spontaneous improvement. That is, they improve without treatment because GO is self-limiting. GO eventually resolves spontaneously although the course of the disease varies as does the need for medical intervention, a subject explored in chapter 10.

3
SIGNS AND SYMPTOMS

The signs and symptoms of GO include a wide variety of characteristic visual signs as well as a cluster of diverse ocular symptoms. "Signs" refers to physical changes that the doctor notes in his or her examination, whereas symptoms refer to the changes that patients experience.

Typical signs include erratic blinking and altered gaze. Typical symptoms include grittiness, tearing, blurring, spastic movements such as staring, proptosis (bulging of the eyeball, exophthalmos), lid retraction, orbital neuropathy, diplopia (double vision), and ocular dryness. Complications or conditions that sometimes occur in GO include ophthalmoplegia (paralysis of the eye muscle, particularly on upward gaze) and compression of the optic nerve. Complications are discussed further in chapter 5.

In GO, ocular findings are most specific or characteristic when they occur bilaterally, affecting both eyes. Certain combinations of signs and symptoms, such as bilateral lid retraction with proptosis and restrictive ophthalmoplegia, are considered virtually diagnostic for GO (meaning that these symptoms are essentially sufficient to diagnose GO), especially in patients with a history of autoimmune thyroid disease. However, signs and symptoms in GO aren't always bilateral. Unilateral symptoms can occur. And because symptoms are often asymmetrical, the eye that is worse may be so prominent that the symptoms may appear unilateral when both eyes are affected.

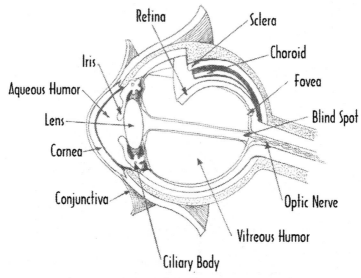

*The Structure of the Eye. Illustrated by Marvin G. Miller. Copyright ©
Elaine A. Moore. Reprinted with permission.*

While the following signs and symptoms help lead to a diagnosis of
GO, some of these indicators are also associated with other disorders,
including myasthenia gravis and certain pseudotumors and tumors.
Chapter 9, which describes how GO is diagnosed, includes a list of other
conditions that can mimic GO and contribute to diagnostic difficulties.

Signs of GO

The signs of GO refer to certain manifestations or traits that are characteristically seen in GO during an eye examination. Certain signs are considered diagnostically significant for GO. The four signs listed below are
the signs most commonly seen in GO:

- Von Graefe's sign: upper eyelid lag on down-gaze.
- Dalrymple's sign: upper eyelid retraction.
- Stellwag's sign: incomplete and infrequent blinking.

- Ballet's sign: palsy or paralysis affecting one or more extraocular muscle.
  The following signs, while not as common, may also occur in GO:

- Abadie's sign: spasms in levator muscle with upper eyelid retraction.
- Boston's sign: uneven, jerky motion of upper eyelid on inferior movement (controlled by the inferior muscles in the rear or posterior of the eye).
- Enroth's sign: edema of the lower eyelid.
- Gellinek's sign: abnormal pigmentation of the upper eyelid.
- Gifford's sign: difficulty in everting (turning outward or inside out) the upper lid.
- Goffroy's sign: absent creases in the forehead on superior gaze (controlled by the superior or front ocular muscles).
- Griffith's sign: lower lid lag on upward gaze.
- Joffroy's sign: absence of normal contraction of the frontalis muscle when looking up.
- Knie's sign: uneven pupil dilation in dim light.
- Means' sign: increased superior scleral show on up-gaze.
- Riesman's sign: bruit (sound of increased blood flow) over eyelid.
- Rosenbach's sign: tremor of the closed lids.
- Vigouroux's sign: eyelid puffiness.

Symptoms of GO

Depending on one's genetic and immunological make-up, as well as their disease progression and thyroid hormone levels, patients with GO may experience one or more of the following symptoms.

Blurred vision

Blurred vision results from alterations of the tear film or from corneal astigmatism (irregularity of the shape of the cornea, which may result from congestive infiltration). Alterations of the tear film may be related to excessive or decreased lacrimation or tearing; blurring caused by either of these causes may be relieved by blinking, although patients with dry eye may require the addition of moisture drops such as artificial tears.

Visual blurring may also be caused by minor degrees of extraocular muscle balance that aren't severe enough to cause diplopia; this form of blurring improves when either eye is closed. The visual blurring of greatest concern persists for days or weeks and continues even when one eye is closed. This type of blurring is often associated with a reduction in color brightness or altered visual quality in one portion of the visual field. This type of blurring can suggest optic neuropathy.

Chemosis

Chemosis refers to edema of the bulbar conjunctiva. The conjunctiva is the mucous membrane that lines the inner surface of the eyelids and extends over the forepart of the eyeball where it becomes the bulbar conjunctiva. Chemosis ultimately causes corneal swelling.

Conjunctival exposure

Conjunctival exposure refers to frank (meaning fully demonstrated) exposure of the delicate conjunctival membrane that lines the eyelids and covers the eyeball in the front of the eye. Extended periods of conjunctival exposure can lead to corneal inflammation (keratitis) or corneal ulceration.

Corneal compromise

The cornea becomes compromised when the eyelids don't offer adequate protection, either because of proptosis or eyelid retraction. Corneal compromise can result in corneal ulceration or exposure keratitis.

Diplopia

Diplopia is a condition of horizontal or vertical double vision caused by restriction of antagonist muscles rather than weakness of the muscles that facilitate movement. Diplopia occurs when the fields of vision overlap. Usually one muscle is restricted and the opposing muscle becomes hyperactive to compensate. Although diplopia is usually intermittent at its onset, occurring most often when the patient is tired, as GO progresses, images separate further apart and diplopia becomes more persistent. Most diplopia in GO is binocular, meaning that it can be corrected when one eye is covered or closed.

Exophoria

Exophoria is a latent form of strabismus in which the visual axes (meaning, the visual lines of vision as opposed to the orbital axes) tend outward toward the temple.

Exophthalmos (Proptosis)

Exophthalmos refers to a bulging or protrusion of the eyeball as the globe is anteriorially (forward) displaced within its socket. Proptosis is generally defined as corneal protrusion, measuring greater than 21 mm or exhibiting asymmetrical measurements (difference between the two eyes) greater than 3 mm when measured with an exophthalmometer. Thyroid eye disease does not cause painful proptosis. Painful proptosis is more commonly associated with lesions resulting from orbital infections, posterior scleritis, pseudotumors, and some orbital tumors.

Exposure keratitis

Exposure keratitis refers to an inflammation of the cornea caused by inadequate lid closure resulting from proptosis or eyelid dysfunction. Untreated, exposure keratitis can progress to ulceration of the cornea, panophthalamitis (inflammation or infection of the entire eye), and visual loss.

Extraocular muscle infiltration

Extraocular muscle infiltration is a condition in which deposits of white blood cells and glycosaminoglycan infiltrate the extraocular muscles, causing a separation of fibers and muscle enlargement. This condition contributes to proptosis as the body attempts to contain the additional fluids and tissue.

Eye motility problems

Eye motility problems are abnormalities in restriction of the eyes, particularly restriction of upward gaze, which may progress to a limitation of horizontal eye movement. Eye motility problems occur as one or more of the extraocular muscles that support the eye become restricted in their movement. Eye motility problems may cause diplopia.

Eyelid retraction

Eyelid retraction is a condition characterized by an inward folding of the eyelid. Eyelid retraction may affect the upper or lower lids of one or both eyes. Early in the course of the disease lid retraction may be due to the exaggerated sympathetic nervous system response seen in hyperthyroidism; in later disease stages, retraction may be caused by fibrosis (scarring or the presence of collagen deposits).

Fibrosis

Fibrosis is a process in which tissues change texture, becoming fibrous or woody, with an appearance similar to that of scar tissue.

Thyroid Eye Disease

Foreign body sensation

Foreign body sensation refers to a condition characterized by the feeling of sand, grit or particles occurring between the eye and eyelid.

Grittiness

Grittiness refers to a condition of eye dryness in which the eyes feel as if they have sand in them.

Heterophoria

Heterophoria is a latent form of strabismus (impaired eye motility) in which one eye tends to deviate either medially or laterally.

Hypertropia

Hypertropia, or upward strabismus, is a condition characterized by elevation of the line of vision of one eye above that of the other.

Lacrimation (Tearing)

While lacrimation or forming tears is a normal process, excessive lacrimation or tearing leads to watery eyes. Tearing occurs when eyes become too dry.

Lid Lag (Lagophthalmos)

Lid lag or lagophthalmos is a condition of incomplete eyelid closure.

Optic neuropathy

Optic neuropathy refers to a condition characterized by damage to the optic nerve causing blurred vision, loss of color vision, and, if untreated, possible blindness.

Photophobia

Photophobia is a condition of light sensitivity. Patients with photobia can relieve their symptoms by wearing tinted lenses whenever they're exposed to light, especially bright light. A characteristic thyroid frown is seen in many patients with photophobia (and occurs as a result of squinting into light over time).

Periorbital edema

Periorbital edema refers to swelling around the eye, including the lid area and beneath the eye. Periorbital edema is caused by insufficient venous circulation and the fluid retention that occurs in congestive GO.

Pain or discomfort

Eye pain is a serious symptom and should always be promptly reported. Discomfort, aching and soreness are more common complaints and frequently occur in patients with proptosis.

Proptosis (Exophthalmos)

Proptosis refers to a bulging or protrusion of the eyeball caused by enlargement of extraocular muscles and tissues. This enlargement leads to crowding of the orbital cavity and a compensatory decompression that causes the eye to be displaced anteriorly or forward.

Ptosis

Ptosis is a condition of upper eyelid drooping that may be related to paralysis of the oculomotor nerve.

Redness

Dilated blood vessels in GO can lead to redness or erythema of the sclera and the conjunctiva.

Staring

A staring appearance is one of the most common presentations of GO; when thyroid hormone levels are high, the stare is intensified because of the heightened sympathetic response, which causes contraction of the levator muscles. Staring can also be caused or exacerbated by fibrosis and scarring of the eyelid levator muscles.

Strabismus

Strabismus is a condition characterized by an inability of the eyes to focus together because of an imbalance in the muscles that control eye movement. Strabismus, which typically causes squinting, may affect one or both eyes.

Superior limbic keratoconjunctivitis (SLK)

Superior limbic keratoconjunctivitis is an inflammatory disorder affecting the conjunctiva. Because this condition is so often seen in GO, all patients with SLK should be tested for thyroid function.

Swelling

Swelling refers to fluid retention. Impaired venous circulation in GO is responsible for edema or swelling.

Thyroid Eye Disease

Visual impairment

Visual impairment may occur as a result of optic nerve damage (compression or infiltration; change of refraction; choroidal folds [see description in chapter 5]); corneal exposure; or as a non-specific complaint.

Visual loss

Visual loss may occur as a consequence of corneal damage, including corneal ulceration, although its most common cause is optic neuropathy.

Usual Findings in GO

Ocular findings are most specific for GO when they occur in both eyes (bilaterally) and in certain combinations, such as bilateral lid retraction with proptosis. Patients with GO frequently have asymmetric symptoms, meaning that one eye is affected more than the other.

Changes in Appearance

While clinically significant signs and symptoms of GO only occur in a small number of patients, many patients experience troubling cosmetic changes. And while these changes may resolve spontaneously after the active disease phase subsides, patients with persistent cosmetic changes must endure these changes until the disease process itself has resolved. When cosmetic treatment is necessary, it generally must be withheld until muscle changes have stabilized and, often, cosmetic surgery includes several separate procedures. In studies of the psychosocial effects of GO, many patients describe these cosmetic changes as the most devastating. While the physical changes that may occur in GO are described in the following section, psychosocial effects of GO are described in chapter 12.

Usually, patients have a combination of different signs and symptoms although one symptom or sign may be predominant. GO commonly causes the upper eyelid or eyelids to rise higher than usual. This causes patients to look angry or appear to have a prominent stare. Patients with mild GO often complain of photophobia (causing them to squint and frown), foreign body sensation, and increased tearing, which is a sign of dry eye. A vertical crease appearing between the eyebrows is known as a thyroid frown and occurs as the forehead muscles tighten in their attempts to accommodate vision.

Other complaints include discomfort when looking up or a generalized restriction of up-gaze. Increased intraocular pressure on up-gaze is also commonly seen in GO. In later stages of the disease, horizontal eye movement may also become limited.

Proptosis develops as the body tries to deal with expanded tissue related to enlarged eye muscles and increased accumulations of orbital fat. Proptosis is generally greater than 22 mm, and the difference between the two eyes is generally greater than 3 mm, causing an asymmetrical appearance.

A generalized tightening of fibers in the levator muscles that raise and lower the eyelids often occurs in GO. This can lead to eyelid retraction. Early in the course of the disease, the effects of excess thyroid hormone on the sympathetic nervous system may cause eyelid retraction. In the later stages of the disease, fibrosis or scarring of eyelid tissues is generally responsible for eyelid retraction. Eyelid retraction may also occur in patients with proptosis as the eyelids are stretched from their normal position.

Dry Eye and Exposure Keratitis

Because of the effects of proptosis and eyelid retraction, the cornea may be exposed for longer periods of time. This loss of protection on the exposed surface of the eye can lead to dryness and a loss of the normal tear film. Eye dryness can lead to tearing, itchiness, grittiness, and foreign body sensation. The eyes may become painful, reddened and watery, especially when they're exposed to the elements. Patients at risk for corneal exposure are advised to avoid wind and to wear protective lenses.

Exposure keratitis (a condition of corneal inflammation) can also occur in patients who experience inadequate lid closure. Untreated, exposure keratitis can progress to corneal ulceration, perforation, inflammation of the entire eye, and loss of vision. Patients with GO may also develop an acquired corneal astigmatism (irregularity of the shape of the cornea). This may cause blurred vision.

Diplopia

Diplopia or double vision can occur because of the eye muscle changes that occur in GO. These changes affect the way the eye muscles normally move together to produce vision. The muscles lose their normal alignment and lose their ability to move the eye coordinately in all directions.

Thyroid Eye Disease

Periorbital Edema

Inflammation in GO may cause puffiness of the eyelids as well as the thin tissue surrounding the eye. This condition, which is known as periorbital edema, is especially noticeable in the morning. Patients with problems of swelling or puffiness are advised to elevate the top of their beds at night. Patients are also advised to drink plenty of fluids since dehydration worsens or exacerbates this condition.

Lacrimal gland involvement

The lacrimal glands of patients with GO frequently show mild tissue infiltration by mononuclear white blood cells and interstitial edema, which is a condition of excess fluid between lacrimal gland cells. Although this finding suggests that the lacrimal glands are affected in GO, the inflammation that occurs in this area does not progress to fibrosis.

Deviations From the Rule

While most patients develop symptoms of GO within 18 months of their thyroid disorder, other patients develop GO many years before or many years after their first symptoms of thyroid disease. And although most patients develop a number of different eye signs and symptoms, some patients may only experience one symptom, such as increased lacrimation or eyelid spasms. And while most patients have symptoms in both eyes (bilateral involvement), in some people only one eye is affected (unilateral involvement). With sophisticated imaging studies, however, often the eye that appears to be unaffected exhibits similar symptoms, only to a lesser degree.

Euthyroid vs Thyroid Related GO

One recent Chinese study conducted by researchers at the First Affiliated Hospital of Beijing Medical University in Beijing compared patients with thyroid disease and GO to patients with euthyroid Graves' disease (no evidence or history of thyroid disease). Patients with euthyroid Graves' disease were found to be more likely to develop diplopia, experience problems closing lids, have limited eyeball movements, corneal involvement, and unilateral proptosis.

The patients with both thyroid disease and GO were more likely to have more serious complications, such as optic nerve involvement. Patients with euthyroid Graves' disease also showed a better response to drug therapy. In follow-up studies of these patients, 61 percent of the euthryoid group developed hyperthyroidism and goiter within 5 months to 3 years. The remaining 39 percent of euthyroid patients showed no signs of thyroid involvement up to 6 years later.

4

CLASSIFYING GO

Many attempts have been made to classify GO according to certain discrete stages. However, not all patients end up moving through each of these stages. And because the congestive form of GO is an autoimmune disorder, its symptoms frequently wax and wane. Symptoms can also be influenced by a plethora of divergent factors, including diet, nutrient deficiencies and stress. The following classifications are commonly used to describe the stages or phases of GO, both as an aid in classifying disease severity during initial diagnosis, determining if there is a need for therapy, and in evaluating response to therapy.

Major Categories of GO

Patients with thyroid related eye disorders can be divided into three major categories:

1. Patients with active vision-threatening symptoms, such as compressive optic neuropathy or corneal ulceration.

2. Patients with active non-vision threatening symptoms, including myopathy, mild exposure keratopathy, congestive signs and symptoms.

3. Patients with chronic, stable symptoms, such as dryness or mild eyelid retraction.

Phases

Thyroid eye diseases generally progress through phases of disease activity. These phases are important when it comes to making treatment decisions. Treatment aimed at reducing congestion is most effective when it's used during the active disease phase.

1. Active (Wet Phase)

The active phase is the inflammatory phase, usually lasting from three to six months although it may persist for as long as three years. The active phase is associated with worsening eye signs and elevated levels of thyroid stimulating immunoglobulins (TSI).

Symptoms of activity include:

A recent change in periorbital appearance or diplopia, photophobia (light sensitivity), excessive watering, and aching orbits sometimes associated with eye movements.

Signs of activity include:

An obvious, fluid-filled distending eyelid, red eyelid, red eye or bright red vessels, and swollen conjunctiva.

2. Plateau Phase (Reduced Activity)

In the plateau phase, the inflammatory process slows down and many patients experience spontaneous improvement. Often, in the plateau phase, patients become unsatisfied with their degree of improvement and impatient for spontaneous improvement to occur. This can be a frustrating time because patients would like to see faster results. However, this isn't the best time to institute therapy because the immune system cells that therapy (steroids and orbital irradiation) targets are no longer active, rendering treatment at this time ineffective.

3. Inactive (Dry or Resolution Phase)

In the inactive phase, the inflammatory disease process subsides. Slowly, this inactive phase may lead to fibrosis if spontaneous resolution does not occur. During the resolution phase, the extraocular muscles may heal by progressive fibrosis, which may cause contractures (permanent muscle shortening) and diplopia. Patients in this phase do not show signs of inflammation, but they may still have exophathlmos, be prone to corneal exposure, and suffer diplopia due to fibrosis or tethering of the extraocular muscles.

Individual Disease Course

The time frame for GO shows considerable variation although most patients will experience a return to normal within 12 months. In a study of 59 patients with mild GO, at initial evaluation, 64 percent experienced improvement within 12 months without specific eye therapy; 22 percent showed no changes; and 14 percent showed disease progression 12 months after the initial evaluation.

NO SPECS

NO SPECS is an acronym adopted by the American Thyroid Association in 1969. Decades ago this system was widely used to describe the classifications or stages of GO, and it was expected that the disease would move through these progressive stages. At the patient's initial eye examination, he or she would be formally classified, and told that the next stages would follow. Even when this system was in use, many ophthalmologists realized that symptoms of later stages could occur before those in earlier stages, and many patients did not move through these stages at all.

Today it is well known that patients do not necessarily pass through these stages, and symptoms attributed to a certain stage in NO SPECS may appear at any time without having symptoms characteristic of earlier stages. Consequently, these classifications were revised in 1974. The original guidelines of NO SPECS are primarily used today to help in classifying GO in terms of no, mild, moderate, or severe disease.

- N (()):   No signs or symptoms present.
- O (I):   Only symptoms of ocular irritation such as dryness or grittiness.
- S (II):   Soft tissue involvement (perioribital edema).
- P (III):   Proptosis.
- E (IV):   Extraocular muscle involvement (ophthalmoplegia).
- C (V):   Corneal involvement (dense punctate epitheliopathy, infiltration and ulceration).
- S (VI):   Sight loss with or without visual field compromise secondary to compressive optic neuropathy.

Classification of GO by Werner

Today, most ophthalmologists find the classification of Graves' ophthalmopathy by Sidney Werner to be more helpful than that of NO SPECS. This is a numbered system, outlined as follows:

1. No symptoms or signs.
2. Signs only, such as upper lid retraction, staring vision, lid lag; no symptoms.
3. Soft tissue involvement (symptoms and signs).
4. Exophthalmos.
    i. Extraocular muscle involvement; includes diplopia.
    ii. Corneal involvement.
    iii. Loss of vision (optic neuropathy).

Criteria of Mourits- The Clinical Activity Score (CAS)

Another widely-used classification system for GO follows the criteria of Mourits and his associates. The criteria of Mourits includes the following parameters, which are used for assessing disease progression or disease activity:

- Spontaneous retrobulbar pain
- Painful oppressive feeling on or behind the globe
- Pain with eye movements, including attempted up, side or down gaze
- Erythema (redness) of the eyes, eyelids or conjunctiva
- Swelling
- Chemosis
- Edema of the eyelids
- Increase in proptosis of 2 mm or more during a period of 1–3 months
- Impaired eye function
- Decrease in visual acuity of 1 or more lines on the Snellen chart (described in chapter 9) using a pinhole during a period of 1–3 months
- Decrease of eye movements in any direction equal to or greater than 5 degrees during an evaluation period of 1–3 months

In this system, which is known as the Clinical Activity Score (CAS), one point is given for any manifestation of disease, with 0 indicating no activity and 10 indicating very high disease activity. After two consecutive clinical examinations an activity score can be determined. According to this classification, patients with scores greater than 3 have active eye disease and show a better response to treatment than those with lower scores.

Classification by an Artificial Neural Network

Researchers in Nova Scotia, Canada recently described an artificial neural network system that classifies GO and predicts progression based on parameters measured at the first clinical examination. Parameters used in this evaluation include: lid fissure measurement; Hertel measurements; color vision assessment; cover test and Hess screen; visual acuity assessment; tonometry; fundus examination; visual field assessment; and orbital computed tomography or ultrasonography to measure soft-tissue changes. See chapter 9 for a description of these procedures.

Thyroid Manager's Classification of the Ocular Changes in Graves' Disease

Thyroid Disease Manger, The Thyroid and its Diseases is an online clinical thyroid textbook written by an international group of endocrinologists who specialize in thyroid disease. Intended for use by physicians, researchers and patients, this text is regularly updated.

In chapter 12, *Complications in Graves' Disease*, the authors offer a system for classifying GO with six major classes and four grades for each class. The classes include:

1. No signs or symptoms.
2. Signs limited to upper lid retraction and stare, with or without lid lag and proptosis.
3. Soft tissue involvement, with symptoms of excessive lacrimation, sandy sensation, retrobulbar discomfort, and photophobia, but not diplopia.
4. Proptosis associated with classes 2 to 6.
5. Extraocular muscle involvement (usually with diplopia).
6. Corneal involvement, primarily due to lagophthalmos.
7. Vision impairment .

The grades, which further define each class, include "0" indicating no symptoms, a) mild or minimal symptoms, b) moderate involvement and c) marked involvement.

How Formal Classifications Help

Classifying GO helps in determining disease severity and in determining if treatment is necessary or is likely to be beneficial. Classifying GO also helps in evaluating treatment. While some systems of classification are reported to have the ability to predict disease progression, there are a number of variables outside of the classification systems that can affect the course of GO, making classifications possibly misleading in terms of prognosis or final outcome.

Classifications in Patients with Thyrotoxicosis

Thyrotoxicosis is a term used to describe the condition caused by the effects of excess thyroid hormone. Nearly all patients with thyrotoxicosis will show signs of GO upon close examination. However, the symptoms caused by excess thyroid hormone are not related to disease activity as they are in the congestive form of GO.

The predominant abnormality in thyrotoxicosis may only be widening of the palpebral fissure, and lag of the globe on upward or downward gaze, causing a pop-eyed appearance. These abnormalities may cause the eye to appear exophthalmic, but measurement may show that there is no actual proptosis.

These symptoms can also occur when patients are administered excess thyroid hormone. In addition to the symptoms mentioned above, the local action of sympathetic stimulation (caused by excess thyroid hormone) on one of the major eyelid muscles—Muller's superior palpebral muscle—will cause spasm and retraction of the upper lid. However, unlike symptoms in congestive GO, the symptoms attributed to thyrotoxicosis abate as thyroid hormone levels return to the normal range. Depending on their degree, symptoms caused by thyrotoxicosis are classified as mild, moderate or severe.

5
ORBITAL ANATOMY & INFLAMMATORY DISEASE

Chapter 5 describes the eye and its structures, showing how the eye's various structures and components work together to create vision. This chapter also describes the changes to eye structures that result from orbital inflammatory disease and explains how changes to the eye's structures may compromise vision.

Anatomy & Physiology, Structure and Function of the Eye

Orbital anatomy refers to the inherent structures—the bones, tissue and fluids—that make up the eye and how these structures are normally situated in relation to one another. The orbit refers to the bony house or cage that covers and protects the eye while the globe refers to the tissues that make up the eye. Physiology refers to the functions of the various structures that comprise the eye, for example, the lacrimal glands producing and secreting tears, which bathe and moisten the globe. Each of the eye's structures has a unique physiological function that contributes to vision.

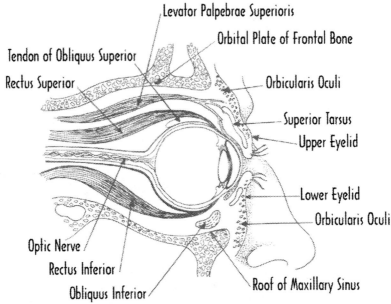

Levator Palpebrae Superioris

Orbital Plate of Frontal Bone

Tendon of Obliquus Superior

Rectus Superior

Orbicularis Oculi

Superior Tarsus

Upper Eyelid

Lower Eyelid

Orbicularis Oculi

Optic Nerve

Rectus Inferior

Obliquus Inferior

Roof of Maxillary Sinus

Sagital Section of Right Orbital Cavity. Illustrated by Marvin G. Miller. Copyright © Elaine A. Moore. Reprinted with permission.

The Key Players

The cornea is the crystal clear dome that covers the front of the eye. Although it may appear to be an invisible film, the cornea serves to refract and bend light. The sclera or "white of the eye" is the eye's tough outer wall, which encloses the eyeball except for the part covered by the cornea. And the choroid is the thin spongy layer of blood vessels situated between the sclera and the retina situated at the back of the eye.

The iris is the part of the eye that gives it its color or pigment. The pupil is the opening in the middle of the iris that allows light to enter the eye. The lens is a body of tissue situated behind the pupil that further refracts light waves and sends them to the retina in the back of the eye. Here, specialized cells known as rods and cones convert the light rays into nerve signals or electrical impulses. These are transported through the optic nerve to the brain where they're interpreted as images. If these signals are unable to reach the brain properly, vision cannot occur.

The Eye and its Structures

The eye consists of the eyeball or globe along with its fluids, glands, and major tissues, such as the cornea and retina. The eye also contains: extraocular muscles; ligaments and tissue expansions that support the globe; a bony cage or orbit that houses the tissues; and eyelids and eyelashes that protect it. The eye also consists of a nervous system that allows it to communicate with other organs, and a vascular system that provides blood circulation, providing oxygen and other nutrients to the cells.

The three layers of the eye

1. The external layer, formed by the sclera and cornea;
2. The intermediate layer, which is divided into 2 parts: an anterior or front that contains the iris and ciliary body, and the posterior or rear section that contains the choroids (a vascular membrane situated between the retina and sclera); and
3. The internal layer, or the sensory part of the eye known as the retina.

The Lens and the Retina

When light strikes the outer layer of the eye's surface, which is known as the cornea, it bends or refracts the incoming light onto the lens. The lens is a spherical, transparent body situated behind the pupil. The lens is suspended in the orbit by ligaments known as zonule fibers. Zonule fibers attach the lens to the anterior or front portion of the ciliary body.

Unlike the cornea, the lens can change its shape and its refractive powers, allowing the eye to change its focal point. The lens further refocuses the incoming rays, ensuring that the rays come to a sharp focus. From the lens, light rays proceed through a clear jelly-like substance known as vitreous, which gives the rays form and shape; the rays then move on to the retina, which is situated at the posterior or back of the eye.

The Retina's Role in Vision

The resulting image on the retina arrives inverted or upside-down. The retina, which constitutes the back two-thirds of the eye, is composed of a layer of light sensing cells. The macula is its most sensitive area and is responsible for critical focusing, such as in reading. In the retina the light rays begin to be translated into vision.

The retina contains millions of rod and cone cells (rods and cones) that convert light rays into electrical impulses. These impulses are sent through the optic nerve to the brain. The fovea—the center of the retina just behind the macula—contains the highest concentration of cone photoreceptors. The lens focuses light rays onto the fovea for direct or forward vision and fine detail.

When the brain receives these impulses from the retina, it interprets them as images. This refractive process is similar to the way in which cameras are able to take pictures. The cornea and lens act much like a camera lens, and the retina can be compared to film. If the image isn't focused properly, the brain receives a blurry image.

The Main Support, The Extraocular Eye Muscles

Orbital anatomy refers to the position of the orbital globe or eyeball relative to the bony socket in which it's housed. The six tiny extraocular muscles that support the orbit originate at Zinn's annulus, a fibrous extension located at the apex of the orbit. The posterior or rear muscles attach at Zinn's annulus, whereas anteriorly, the muscles insert onto the sclera. The extraocular muscles rotate the eyeball in the orbits and allow the image to be constantly focused on the fovea of the central retina.

The visual axis and the orbital axis are not precisely parallel. The superior rectus muscles elevate and rotate the eye inwardly, and the inferior rectus muscles lower and rotate the eye outwardly. Two oblique muscles run posteriorly to their attachment on the eye. The superior obliques depress, abduct, and rotate the eyes inwardly whereas the inferior oblique muscles elevate, abduct and rotate the eyes outwardly. Another set of muscles, the medial and lateral rectus muscles, are straightforward abductors and adductors respectively.

The extraocular muscles are connected by a fibrous sheath of connective tissue that coalesces between muscles, creating a boundary between the eye's intraconal (within the area housing cone cells) compartment and the extraconal space surrounding the cones.

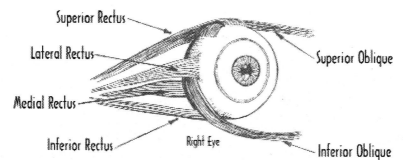

*The Extraocular Muscles. Illustrated by Marvin G. Miller. Copyright ©
Elaine A. Moore. Reprinted with permission.*

How Extraocular Muscles Contribute to Vision

The extraocular muscles work together to move the eye, allowing for
vision. The four rectus muscles control the eye's movements from left to
right and up and down. The two oblique muscles rotate the eyes inward
and outward.

These six muscles work in unison to move the eye. As one of the ocular muscles contracts, the opposite muscle in that eye relaxes. This allows
for smooth, precise eye movements. Furthermore, the muscles of both
eyes work in unison to ensure that the eyes are always aligned.

Individual Extraocular Muscles

1. *Medial Rectus*: The medial rectus muscle rotates the eye inward
   towards the nose. This movement is known as adduction.
2. *Lateral Rectus*: The lateral rectus muscle rotates the eye towards the
   temple. This movement is known as abduction outward.
3. *Inferior Rectus*: The inferior rectus muscle is the primary muscle. It's
   responsible for turning the eye in a downward direction, a movement
   known as depression.
4. *Superior Rectus*: The superior rectus muscle is the primary muscle
   responsible for turning the eye upward. This movement is known as
   elevation.
5. *Inferior Oblique*: The inferior oblique muscle rotates the eye upward
   and outward towards the temple. This movement is known as
   extorsion.

6. *Superior Oblique*: The superior oblique rotates the eye both downward and inward towards the nose. This movement is known as intorsion.

Extraocular Muscle Changes in GO

Although the extraocular muscles are usually enlarged in GO, the muscle fibers remain normal. Muscle enlargement is not due to enlargement of individual fibers. It is due to the separation of muscle fibers caused by fluids and fatty deposits, the mucinous (jelly-like) substance glycosaminoglycan, fibrosis or scar tissue, and by aggregates or clusters of white blood cells. While most patients with GO exhibit enlargement of the superior rectus muscle, almost as many patients exhibit enlargement of the medial rectus muscle or the inferior rectus muscle. Any of the six extraocular muscles may become enlarged in GO.

Crowding in The Orbital Cavity

Normally, the bony orbital cavity that houses the eye holds approximately 26 ml of tissue and fluids. The anterior or front portion of the cavity contains the globe, and the posterior or rear portion contains the extraocular muscles. Proptosis occurs when the contents of the orbital cavity exceed the usual volume, displacing the contents and pushing them forward. The average muscle volume is normally 3.0 to 6.8 ml, and the volume of orbital fat and connective tissue is 8.2 to 14.0 ml. In patients with proptosis, muscle volume may be as high as 21.0 ml and the volume of orbital fat and connective tissue may be as high as 22 ml.

The Cornea

The cornea is the eye's outermost layer. Appearing as a clear, dome-shaped surface, the cornea covers the front of the eye. Although it appears clear, the cornea is composed of a highly organized group of cells and proteins. However, the cornea has no blood vessels to nourish it or to offer protection against infection. Instead, it receives nourishment from tears and from the aqueous humor (vitreous humor) that fills the chamber behind it. The cornea must remain transparent to refract light properly.

The cornea also acts as a filter. It screens out some of the most damaging, ultraviolet (UV) wavelengths in sunlight. This protects the lens and retina to possible injury from UV radiation. When the cornea is injured by minor injuries or abrasions, healthy cells migrate to the area and patch the injury. However, if the abrasion or lesion penetrates the cornea too deeply, the healing process takes longer. And the lesion can lead to corneal scarring. This can cause a haze on the cornea that greatly impairs vision.

The Cornea's Layers

The corneal tissue can be divided into five distinct layers, each with its own functions. The layers include:

The Epithelium

The epithelium is the cornea's outermost layer. It comprises about ten percent of the tissue's thickness. This layer, which is composed of epithelial cells, functions to block foreign material from entering the eye and provides a smooth surface that absorbs oxygen and cell nutrients from tears. These nutrients are subsequently distributed to the rest of the cornea. Because the epithelium contains many nerve endings, it is subject to pain. The foundation upon which the other epithelial cells rest is known as the basement membrane.

Bowman's Layer

The Bowman's layer is a transparent sheet of tissue that lies directly below the basement membrane of the epithelium. Primarily composed of collagen, the Bowman's layer can form a scar as it heals from injury. If large and centrally located, these scars can cause vision loss.

Stroma

The stroma, which lies beneath the Bowman's layer, comprises about 90 percent of the cornea's thickness. It primarily consists of water and collagen and is free of blood vessels. The collagen's unique shape, arrangement and spacing are essential in producing the cornea's light-conducting transparency.

Descemet's Membrane

Descemet's membrane, a thin, strong sheet of tissue, lies beneath the stroma. It serves as a protective barrier, protecting against infection and injuries. Descemet's membrane is primarily composed of collagen, which is produced by the endothelial cells that lie below it.

Endothelium

The endothelium is the extremely thin, innermost layer of the cornea. The endothelium is essential for keeping the cornea clear. Normally, fluid leaks slowly from the inside of the eye, moving into the stroma. The endothelium pumps this excess fluid out of the stroma. Otherwise the stroma would swell with water, become hazy and ultimately become opaque. In a healthy eye, there is a perfect balance between the fluid moving in and out of the cornea.

The Oculomotor Nerve

The oculomotor nerve (parasympathetic nerve) innervates the extraocular muscles and the smooth muscles within the eye. This nerve connects with all the eye muscles except the superior oblique and the lateral rectus. Therefore, it helps to elevate, depress and adduct the eyeball. The oculomotor nerve is also responsible for papillary light and accommodation reflexes.

The Optic Nerve

The optic nerve transmits electrical impulses from the retina to the brain, where the image is translated and perceived in an upright position. In congestive GO, the optic nerve may be compressed because of crowding in the orbital cavity. If the compression is severe, the optic nerve's integrity may be compromised and vision may be threatened.

The optic nerve and the central retinal vessels enter the back of the eye at the disc or blind spot.

The Tear Film & Dry Eye

Tears are the eye's primary source of moisture. Tears are continuously produced and drained in the normal healthy eye. Tears keep the eyes moist, help wounds heal, and protect the eye from infection.

The tear film consists of three layers: 1) an outer, oily (lipid) layer that keeps tears from evaporating too quickly and helps tears coat the surface of the eye; 2) a middle (aqueous) layer that nourishes the cornea and conjunctiva; and 3) a bottom (mucin) layer that helps to spread the aqueous layer across the eye to ensure that the eye remains wet.

A condition of dry eye occurs when the eyes produce insufficient fluid. The main symptom is usually a scratchy or sandy feeling, or a feeling that a foreign body is in the eye. Other symptoms include sting-ing or burning, a feeling of heavy eyelids, blurred or changing vision, episodes of excess tearing or lacrimation, a stringy discharge from the eye, pain, and redness.

Dry eye can develop or be aggravated by dry climates, dehydration and by the use of certain medications, particularly antihistamines, nasal decongestants, tranquilizers and antidepressant medications. Dry eye may occur as a symptom in thyroid related eye disorders and in the autoimmune disorders rheumatoid arthritis and Sjögren's syndrome.

Pathology of GO

Effects of Muscle Enlargement

Pathology is a term that refers to the disease process and also the struc-tural and functional changes caused by disease. The most characteristic pathologic finding is enlargement of the extraocular muscles. Even slight enlargement can lead to edema (fluid retention) of the fatty and muscu-lar orbital tissues, causing puffiness of the tissues surrounding the eyes. In orbital edema, the lids and periorbital (surrounding the eye) tissues are irritated, injected (congested), and characteristically swollen and puffy. The swollen lids generally feel firm and show no evidence of pitting. The scleral conjunctiva or inner rim of the eye may also appear swollen. In some instances, edematous swollen conjunctiva may protrude beyond the palpebral fissure, which is the space between the margins of the eyelids.

The major radiographic (imaging study) finding in GO is the swollen extraocular muscles, but not their tendons. In contrast, in other condi-tions causing orbital muscle inflammation (such as myositis), the muscle bellies (meaning, the enlarged fleshy body of a muscle) as well as the ten-dons are swollen. Upon physical examination, the insertion of the swollen lateral rectus muscle is often visible as a beefy red area at the inner and outer canthus (angle formed by meeting of lower and upper eyelids) when the patient turns the eye laterally or medially. Normally the muscle insertion is barely visible and is pale pink. In tumors that may be responsible for proptosis, the red area is not seen.

Orbital Congestion and Proptosis

Other pathologic changes in GO include inflammation. Inflammation results from the infiltration or clustering of white blood cells and chemical deposits into orbital tissue. This causes increases in orbital fat that ultimately lead to orbital congestion. Orbital congestion may cause excessive lacrimation or tearing and photophobia (light sensitivity). The eyes may also feel irritated, gritty and sore. As the globe becomes displaced anteriorly (pushed forward), proptosis develops. Normally, the anterior border of the cornea doesn't protrude more than 20 mm beyond the lateral margin of the orbit. When the globe measures 2 to 3 mm beyond this limit, proptosis is present. There are, however, ethnic differences that must be considered when measuring proptosis. Asians have an upper limit of 18 mm of protrusion as measured from the lateral orbital rim, compared with 20 mm for Caucasians, and 22 mm for African Americans.

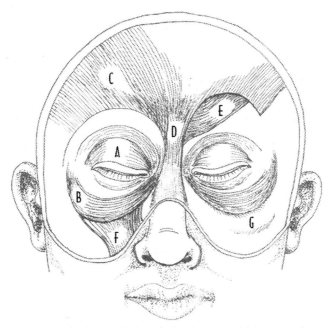

A. Orbicularis Muscle (Palpebral Portion) — eyelid closing muscle
B. Orbicularis Muscle (Orbital Portion) — eyelid closing muscle
C. Frontalis Muscle — forehead muscle
D. Procerus Muscle — muscle that lowers brows
E. Corrugator Muscle — muscle that brings brows together
F. Midfacial Muscles — muscles of the cheek
G. Suborbicularis Fat (SOOF) — fat pad beneath the orbicularis muscle

Thyroid Orbitopathy. Illustrated by Marvin G. Miller. Copyright © Elaine A. Moore. Reprinted with permission.

Strabisumus

Paralysis of the extraocular muscles may also occur in advanced orbital congestion. Upward gaze is affected first and is usually more serious. Loss of convergence or muscle alignment is common and may lead to diplopia. Strabismus is the inability of one eye to attain binocular vision with the other because of imbalance of the extraocular muscles. Muscle paralysis may be severe when exophthalmos is minimal or absent.

Fibrosis

In the more advanced stages of GO, changes include infiltration of the tissue by other immune system cells, including lymphocytes, mast cells, plasma cells, and macrophages. If the disease process continues, this stage is followed by fibrosis, which is characterized by scar tissue and collagen deposits. Often, the scarred and fibrotic muscle causes a fixed strabismus or extraocular muscle imbalance that persists indefinitely unless the problem is surgically corrected.

Increased Intraocular Pressure (IOP)

About 25 percent of patients with GO, especially those with the congestive form of the disorder, develop increased intraocular pressure. In two clinical studies it was shown that an increase in intraocular pressure upon up-gaze correlated with disease severity. Patients who have GO related to abnormal thyroid hormone levels do not develop IOP.

Potential Complications

While most symptoms of GO resolve when thyroid hormone levels are returned to the normal range, the symptoms associated with the congestive form of GO are usually more severe. Blurred vision or ocular pain in patients with GO should be considered an endocrine emergency because of the potential complications. Blurred vision may indicate optic neuropathy, the onset of strabismus or a thinning of the eye's keratin layer, causing a condition known as exposure keratopathy.

Optic Neuropathy

Approximately three to five percent of patients with GO end up developing optic neuropathy. When optic neuropathy occurs, urgent treatment is necessary. Corticosteroids, which offer prompt reduction of inflammation, are the mainstay for this disorder. Nearly all patients with optic neuropathy demonstrate congestive signs and symptoms, including peri-orbital edema, chemosis, vague orbital discomfort, eyelid retraction and muscle inflammation with or without diplopia. The severity of these signs, however, is not related to the severity of the optic neuropathy because any increase in orbital volume can also induce these symptoms.

As previously mentioned, patients with minimal proptosis who are unable to spontaneously decompress are at increased risk. The cause of optic neuropathy in Graves' disease is considered to be a direct compression of the optic nerve by the enlarged extraocular muscles, which are housed within the narrow bony confines of the orbital apex. This compression may be caused by actively inflamed muscles or result from resistant fibrotic muscles located at the orbital apex. Compression directly causes optic nerve injury. Untreated, this can lead to visual loss.

Although the increases in orbital fat volume and muscle volume are increased in overt proptosis, these increases don't usually cause optic neuropathy. Most patients with optic neuropathy show crowding of the orbital apex by enlarged extraocular muscles that surround the optic nerve at the position where it enters the optic canal.

Corneal Exposure

The cornea is the clear layer of tissue that covers the eye. Proptosis may be so severe that patients are unable to close their eyes shut, leaving their cornea permanently exposed. It's not uncommon for such patients to have to administer artificial tears or gels over their corneas throughout the day and tape their eyes such at night to prevent dryness, corneal injury, and ulceration.

Even with protective measures, corneal exposure can result in keratitis or frank ulceration—conditions that cause visual loss, pain, photophobia, tearing, and possibly loss of the eye itself. Proptosis, eyelid retraction and lagophthalmos (lid lag) can all interfere with the patient's efforts to keep a continuous, smooth tear film over the corneal surface.

As a consequence, the corneal surface becomes irregular, causing blurred vision that can vary with each blink. When corneal exposure is significant, superficial punctate (meaning, having tiny pinpoint lesions) cellular defects can be seen by slit-lamp microscopic examination, particularly along the inferior cornea. Loss of corneal epithelial cells in these patients may lead to an infectious keratitis with excavation of the corneal stroma and cellular infiltration. True corneal ulceration usually presents with accompanying conjunctival injection, pain, and photophobia.

Similar, but less severe complaints of tearing and foreign body sensation suggest the possibility of exposure keratopathy, a non-inflammatory eye disease.

Progressive Exophthalmos

When exophthalmos progresses rapidly and becomes a major concern in patients with GO, it is called progressive exophthalmos. If this rapidly progressive condition becomes severe, it's known as malignant exophthalmos.

Exophthalmic Ophthalmoplegia

Ophthalmoplegia refers to a paralysis of the extraocular muscles caused by a muscle restriction. The term exophthalmic ophthalmoplegia refers to the ocular muscle weakness that results in impaired upward gaze. Ophthalmoplegia usually affects one eye and may cause paralysis of the upward gaze. Exophthalmos may be unilateral in the early stage, but this condition usually progresses to bilateral involvement.

6
THE HEART OF THE MATTER,
CELLULAR CHANGES IN GO

While most people think of GO as causing proptosis or eyelid retraction, the underlying cellular changes that lead to these events may have other consequences. In most instances, cellular eye changes can be observed with diagnostic imaging studies but these changes do not cause symptoms. In fact, nearly all patients with Graves' disease will show evidence of cellular changes but will not go on to develop clinically significant GO. And rarely, cellular changes may induce structural orbital changes, which do not alter the eye's appearance although they may interfere with vision.

As we learned in chapter 5, the extraocular muscles in congestive GO become swollen and enlarged, although the muscle fibers are usually normal. Microscopic studies have shown edema, infiltration of white blood cells, primarily lymphocytes and monocytes, deposits of glycosaminoglycan (GAG) and fibrosis or scar tissue. Various immunoglobulins (the proteins from which antibodies are made), including TSH receptor autoantibodies, may also be present.

Muscle enlargement is caused by a separation of muscle fibers. Ground substances, including the substances noted above, lodge between muscle fibers causing this separation. Orbital fibroblast cells and endothelial cells express the immune system markers known as HLA-DR molecules, indicating that immune system genes may contribute to disease development. HLA-DR marker molecules are immune system proteins that cause susceptibility to or protection from certain autoimmune diseases. The expression of these markers on orbital cells suggests immune system involvement in the disease process.

The Target: Orbital Fibroblasts

In GO, orbital fibroblast cells are targeted by both stimulating and blocking TSH receptor antibodies. TSH receptor antibodies cause fibroblasts to deviate from their normal maturation, ultimately causing the autoimmune, congestive form of GO. Fibroblasts are immature cells that eventually develop, as needed, into various cell lines. The destiny of orbital fibroblasts, which are immature precursor cells found in the eye, is to develop into intermediary cells called preadipocytes. These cells normally mature into orbital tissue cells. Under certain circumstances, including activation by TSH receptor antibodies, preadipocytes are directed to become a different type of cell called an adipocyte. As adipocytes, these cells express TSH receptor protein and they produce excess amounts of glycosaminoglycan (GAG), the mucinous substance found in congestive GO.

Immune System Changes

The primary immune system cells are white blood cells known as lymphocytes. Two primary subtypes of lymphocytes exist: T lymphocytes scout for foreign antigens and become activated when they encounter foreign antigens or inappropriately recognize self-antigens as if they were foreign. B lymphocytes react to activated T lymphocytes and go on to produce antibodies and autoantibodies.

According to current theory, T lymphocytes that are TSH reactive (meaning they lead to the development of TSH receptor antibodies) may seek out orbital fibroblast cells that express TSH receptor protein, setting the stage for the development of congestive GO. The immune system cells that infiltrate orbital tissue also produce potent chemicals known as cytokines. Cytokines, which are described further in this chapter as well as in chapter 7, also influence the development and course of GO.

Microscopic examination of orbital tissue in GO shows intense infiltration of orbital tissue by mononuclear (white blood cells with a single nucleus) inflammatory cells, particularly lymphocytes, plasma cells, macrophages and mast cells.

TSH Receptor Antibodies

It is widely accepted today that the same TSH receptor antibodies (TRAb) that cause thyroid dysfunction in autoimmune thyroid disease cause the development of GO. There are three subtypes of TRAb: stimulating, blocking and binding antibodies. Stimulating TSH receptor antibodies (also known as thyroid stimulating immunoglobulins or TSI) are well known for reacting with TSH receptors on thyroid cells and causing excess thyroid hormone production. TSI are the cause of hyperthyroidism in Graves' disease. Blocking antibodies prevent TSH from reacting with the TSH receptor, causing hypothyroidism. Binding antibodies (TBII) include TSI and other antibodies that bind with inert epitopes or binding areas on the TSH receptor.

Most patients with autoimmune thyroid disease have a combination of different types of TRAb. The antibody that predominates determines what disease the patient will have, with TSI predominating in Graves' disease, and blocking TRAb predominating in patients with Hashimoto's thyroiditis. The particular combination of TRAb that a patient has also plays a role in whether he or she will develop GO.

Korean researchers have demonstrated that Graves' disease patients who have both TSI and blocking TSH receptor antibodies are most likely to develop GO. Their study indicated that only patients with blocking TRAb were at risk for developing GO.

Researchers in the Netherlands support this finding. In studies conducted in Amsterdam, researchers have demonstrated that TSH receptor antibodies correlate directly with the Clinical Activity Score of Mourits. These studies support the theory that TSH receptor antibodies react with TSH receptor protein expressed on orbital cells in GO.

TPO Antibodies

Thyroid peroxidase (TPO) antibodies are another type of thyroid antibody. TPO antibodies, which primarily act by destroying thyroid cells, are primarily seen in hypothyroidism, although they may occur in up to 88 percent of patients with Graves' disease. Their role in the development of GO is largely unknown and may be coincidental. There are many conflicting studies, some indicating that TPO antibodies have an association with GO, and some showing that patients with high titers of TSI and no TPO antibodies are most likely to develop GO. The general consensus is that their role in GO is largely unknown although they may contribute to specific symptoms when they are present. They are not considered to be the underlying cause of GO.

Retrobulbar Tissue

One of the hallmarks of GO is the swelling of retrobulbar tissue. This swelling is primarily caused by excessive secretion of GAGs, the mucinous chemical substances produced by adipocytes. Biopsies of affected extraocular muscles show a marked expansion of the endomysial space. This is directly caused by an increased number of collagen fibers interspersed with a granular amorphous deposits of hyaluronic acid, the predominant type of GAG. Because of its affinity for water, GAG accumulations directly lead to orbital edema and tissue expansion.

Cytokine Expression

Cytokines are immune system chemicals produced by white blood cells during the inflammatory immune response. The most well known cytokines are the interleukins, interferons, tumor necrosis factor and various growth factors. Cytokines are able to exert different effects on the body's cells depending on the situation (i.e., toxins, injury, response to foreign antigens, etc.), as they work to control the severity of the immune response.

Studies show that in active GO, patients show higher blood levels of IL-2, IL-6, and TNF when compared to normal persons. This shows that several different cytokines participate in both the occurrence and development of GO. Current research in GO as well as a number of other autoimmune disorders is directed at therapies designed to block cytokine production.

7

THE AUTOIMMUNE ELEMENT

While many people with GO have eye changes related to abnormal thyroid hormone levels, the congestive form of Graves' ophthalmopathy is considered to be an autoimmune disease distinct from the autoimmune thyroid disorders with which it is commonly associated. The same stimulating TSH receptor antibodies (also known as thyroid stimulating immunoglobulin or TSI) that cause hyperthyroidism in Graves' disease cause the congestive infiltrative form of GO. Chapter 7 describes the immune system and explains the immune system changes that lead to the congestive autoimmune form of GO.

Autoimmune Thyroid Disease

Autoimmune thyroid diseases (AITDs) are diseases caused by an immune system defect that produces thyroid autoantibodies that target thyroid tissue. Certain thyroid antibodies destroy thyroid cells, while others cause thyroid cells to produce excess thyroid hormone. AITDs include a number of different conditions, the most common being autoimmune hypothyroidism (Hashimoto's thyroiditis) and autoimmune hyperthyroidism (Graves' disease). In the autoimmune thyroid disorder Hashitoxicosis, people with Hashimoto's thyroiditis also have the thyroid stimulating immunoglobulins (TSI) responsible for hyperthyroidism in Graves' disease.

Consequently, although patients with Hashitoxicosis are primarily hypothyroid, they experience transient symptoms of hyperthyroidism. People with AITD may have Hashimoto's thyroiditis, Graves' disease and Hashitoxicosis at different times in one lifetime, depending on the type of thyroid antibodies that are predominant at the time. In some instances, when patients who appear euthyroid are tested for thyroid antibodies, they are found to have Hashitoxicosis. This chapter describes the role of the immune system in producing thyroid antibodies, and explains how these antibodies cause the development of congestive GO.

The Immune System

The immune system is a constellation of diverse bodily organs and cells that work together to protect us from foreign substances called foreign antigens. The key players are the immune system's white blood cells (leukocytes). Most antigens are protein molecules, although they may also be carbohydrates or lipids. Common foreign antigens that white blood cells guard against include pollen, bacterial and viral particles, food particles, toxins and dander.

Depending on their genetic make-up, including immune system genes and markers, most people will react to some but not all foreign antigens. A person's individual genetic make-up also determines how strongly he or she will react to these antigens. Human leukocyte antigen (HLA) markers on white blood cells control the immune system's reactions to antigens. Individuals with certain HLA markers are susceptible to developing certain autoimmune disorders.

Immune System Organs

The bone marrow and thymus are the human body's primary immune system organs because they are necessary for the production, maturation and storage of white blood cells. The key players, the immune system white blood cells known as lymphocytes, originate in the bone marrow. A certain type of white blood cell known as the T lymphocyte migrates to the thymus. Here, T lymphocytes mature and learn their specific functions, that is, what antigens they should react with. Normally, any cells programmed to react with the body's own tissue (self antigens) are destroyed in the thymus.

Secondary immune system organs, which serve to store lymphocytes until they're needed, include the spleen, tonsils, adenoids, appendix, lymph nodes, lymph fluid, the skin, and certain patches of tissue that line the alimentary tract. These discrete patches, which are found in the respiratory tract and digestive tract, protect us if we happen to ingest toxic substances.

Immune System Cells

Immune system cells include a variety of different white blood cells. The most important immune system players are the lymphocytes. The lymphocyte family has several different subsets. The primary subsets are the helper and suppressor lymphocytes. The most important lymphocytes are the T helper cells because they initiate the immune reaction whereas T suppressor and natural killer (NK) lymphocytes help destroy cancerous cells, toxic cells and cells that become autoreactive. Autoreactive T lymphocyte cells ultimately cause the production of autoantibodies unless they are destroyed by suppressor lymphocytes. People with autoimmune diseases generally have a deficient number of suppressor lymphocytes, which allows autoreactive T lymphocytes cells to initiate autoantibody production.

Antibodies

When T lymphocytes react with foreign antigens they initiate a series of steps that lead to the production of antibodies. Antibodies are made from proteins known as immunoglobulins, and serve to protect us from foreign antigens. For instance, if we're exposed to measles, we develop specific antibodies that protect us from contracting measles from a subsequent exposure. Normally, the human body contains a supply of antibody molecules 100 million times greater than the number of its immune system cells. And normally, the body contains thousands of different types of antibodies.

Autoantibodies

Sometimes, in its scurry to produce the millions of different antibodies it is capable of producing, the immune system errs and produces antibodies against self-components or self-antigens (autoantigens). Self-components are protein particles that belong in the body, such as certain protein particles that reside within our thyroid cells. The antibodies that our immune system inadvertenly produces, which are directed against the tissues and cells of the body are known as autoantibodies. Autoantibodies specifically react with a certain type of protein autoantigen. In the cases of thyroid disease and of GO, TSH receptor antibodies (actually autoantibodies) are directed against a specific protein known as a TSH receptor. The TSH receptor is found in thyroid cells and in orbital cells. When they react with thyroid cells, TSH receptor antibodies cause thyroid cells to produce excess thyroid hormone; when they react with immature orbital fibroblast cells, the cells become adipocytes, cells that produce GAG deposits and collagen, rather than normal orbital cells.

When TSH receptor antibodies react with TSH receptor protein on thyroid cells, these antibodies cause autoimmune thyroid disease. When they react with the cells in our eyes, they cause the congestive autoimmune form of Graves' ophthalmopathy.

T Lymphocytes

The lymphocytic infiltrate (described in chapter 5) in GO is primarily composed of T helper and suppressor lymphocytes along with a few B lymphocytes. Homing of T cells to the orbital fibroblasts in GO (i.e., when the T cells seek out and react with the TSH receptor protein on these orbital fibroblast cells) is facilitated by the expression of HLA-DR antigens (present in most people with Graves' disease and Hashimoto's thyroiditis) and proteins known as adhesion molecules, which are present in orbital endothelial cells.

Cytokine Influences

The tendency for T lymphocytes to infiltrate orbital tissue is also enhanced by the cytokines interleukin (IL)- 1α, tumor necrosis factor (IFN)-α, interferon (IFN)-γ, and Graves immunoglobulin G (TSH receptor antibodies). This means that the abnormal concentration of cytokines in patients with GO influences what antigens T lymphocytes will seek out. The abnormal cytokine concentrations encourage the T lymphocytes to seek out orbital fibroblast cells that express HLA-D, facilitating the development of congestive GO.

Orbital Fibroblasts

All of the body's cells originate from immature cells known as blast cells. As blast cells mature, they differentiate into various types of tissue cells. Fibroblasts are flat, elongated immature cells destined to become connective tissue cells. Fibroblasts, depending on their location within the body, normally mature to form orbital cells, skin cells and bone cells.

During the immune response that leads to and perpetuates GO, T lymphocytes rush to orbital tissue, seeking out orbital fibroblast cells that express HLA-DR. These lymphocytes also release a variety of different cytokines during the immune response. A number of cytokines, described later in this chapter, cause orbital fibroblasts to step up their production of glycosaminoglycan (GAG). GAG deposits then aggregate between the fibers of extraocular muscles, causing muscle enlargement.

The Immune Response

Viewed through a microscope, the immune response is a subject of great drama. The immune system initiates a response whenever it is threatened by foreign antigens or responds to self antigens as if they were foreign antigens. The key players, the T lymphocytes, multiply and divide during the immune response, increasing their numbers. Then they rush to the site of attack. Here, they crowd the area, causing a condition known as lymphocytic infiltration. In GO, this is demonstrated by the deposits of GAG and lymphocytes that infiltrate the spaces between muscle fibers. In addition, T lymphocytes release cytokines and other immune system chemicals known as complement molecules. These chemicals launch their own plan of attack by causing cell growth and cell destruction, depending on what specific antigen they're reacting to. The immediate effects of the immune response include inflammation and sometimes fever, mechanisms designed to protect the body from a foreign antigen attack. In GO, the process leads to inflammation and congestive infiltration, and the process persists as long as TSH receptor antibodies are available to react with TSH receptor expressed on orbital fibroblast cells. Thus, the active stage of GO is characterized by high blood levels of TSH receptor antibodies.

GAG Production

The autoimmune response in GO involves increased production of GAG by orbital fibroblasts. This mucinous material forms deposits in retrobulbar tissue. Orbital connective tissue in patients with GO contains an average of 254 mcg GAG per gram of wet tissue. Normal control subjects contain an average of 150 mcg GAG per gram of wet tissue. In some systems used to evaluate the active stage of GO, elevated blood levels of GAG are used as a positive marker for active GO.

The GAG family includes a number of different chemicals, the primary one being hyaluronic acid. All of the GAG subtypes contain polyanionic charges, which cause them to attract and bind large amounts of water. (Incidentally, GAG is the material that lodges beneath the skin in myxedema, giving the skin a waterlogged, swollen appearance.)

Thyroglobulin

Thyroglobulin is a large molecular weight protein produced by the thyroid gland. Normally, it is only found in the thyroid gland. A high serum thyroglobulin level reflects physical damage or inflammation to the gland in which case thyroglobulin leaks into the circulation. Researchers in Italy have found thyroglobulin to be present in the orbital tissues of patients with GO, suggesting that thyroglobulin transported through the lymphatic system may contribute to the development of GO.

Autoimmune Contributions

The Elusive Target Antigen

The protein known as the TSH receptor normally can be found on the surface of thyroid cells. Here, it is normally stimulated by the hormone thyrotropin (also known as thyroid stimulating hormone or TSH) to produce adequate amounts of thyroid hormone to serve the body's needs. For years, researchers tried to determine what component of orbital cells served as the target antigen. In recent years, researched have learned that TSH receptor protein expressed on orbital cells is the target in GO.

TSH receptor autoantibodies (TRAb) react with the TSH receptor found on the surface of orbital cells, generating an autoimmune response, complete with lymphocytic infiltration and increased GAG production. Studies from the Netherlands show a direct correlation between the clinically active score in GO and the titer of antibodies in the blood.

However, Korean researchers were unable to obtain the same results. This may be explained by the fact that in the initial disease process, TSH receptor antibodies, which are produced by lymphocytes in orbital tissue, are bound to TSH receptor protein in orbital tissue. In the disease process, the lymphocytes keep producing these antibodies. As IgG immunoglobulins, TRAb eventually break down into amino acids. It's likely that TRAb only begin to spill into the blood circulation at a certain critical point, for instance when they're beginning to break down, or when their concentration in orbital tissue reaches a certain maximum amount. It is also unclear whether the Korean researchers measured total TRAb or merely stimulating TRAb (TSI). A number of other studies show that blocking as well as stimulating and binding TRAb are elevated in the blood of patients of GO.

More evidence for the interaction of TRAb and orbital TSH protein as a determinant in GO comes from animal experiments. The first attempts to establish an animal model of Graves' disease involved mice treated with TSH receptor-primed cells. Mice with immune system genes typically seen in GD developed GO, whereas the other mice didn't. The activity of certain cytokines was also consistent with what is seen in humans who develop GO.

More Evidence for the TSH Receptor Target Antigen

Support for this theory can also be found in studies showing that symptoms of GO increase as levels of TSI increase in patients with untreated Graves' disease. In one study of GO patients who had been euthyroid for two months, a direct relationship was observed between serum TSH receptor antibody levels and quantitative measures of GO, such as proptosis and the clinical activity score.

Levels of TSI, and sometimes blocking TSH receptor antibodies, are also known to increase after radioiodine ablation for Graves' disease. The incidence of GO increases significantly in patients after RAI as their levels of TRAb rise.

Therapeutic Implication of Cytokines

Certain cytokines stimulate orbital fibroblasts cells to become adipocytes, cells that produce GAG, rather than orbital tissue cells. The severity of GO is thought to be influenced by the specific cytokines (interleukin 1 beta, transforming growth factor beta, fibroblast growth factors and interleukin 6), which promote the production of adipocytes; and interferon gamma and TGF-beta, which inhibit the production of adipocytes. Manipulating the levels of these cytokines is one of the goals of researchers who are working to develop effective treatments for GO.

Monoclonal antibody treatment is one way of manipulating cytokine levels. By administering antibodies that are synthetically produced to react with certain cytokines, these cytokines can be inactivated or destroyed. Monoclonal therapy is already widely used in other autoimmune disorders such as Crohn's disease.

8
RISK FACTORS

While certain symptoms in GO are directly related to abnormal thyroid hormone levels, the congestive form of GO is known to be influenced by various risk factors, including smoking and diet. Similar to most autoimmune diseases, the congestive autoimmune form of GO is caused by a combination of genetic and environmental factors. That is, individuals with certain immune system genes are predisposed to developing GO when they are exposed to certain environmental factors, particularly stress, excess dietary iodine, saturated fats and sugar. Both stress and excess iodine cause immune system changes that encourage the production of thyroid antibodies, whereas saturated fats and sugars cause immune system changes that promote inflammation. Chapter 8 describes the genetic influences that predispose individuals to developing GO and the environmental factors that trigger and exacerbate GO.

Genetic Influences

The genetics of GO are poorly understood. To date, there is no one gene that predisposes individuals to developing GO. According to current theory, individuals with GO have certain genes that predispose them to developing GO when they're exposed to certain environmental triggers.

HLA Genes
Human leukocyte antigen (HLA) genes are immune system genetic markers found on the short arm of chromosome six in humans. HLA genes determine what substances our immune system will react with and how intense this immune response will be. Many autoimmune conditions

have an association with certain HLA genes. For instance, most patients with Graves' disease have HLA antigens A1, DR3 and B8. However, the link for HLA genes and GO is not as strong as it is for Graves' disease. Researchers in Japan have found that GO occurs more often in patients with HLA DQW3.

A recent study of patients with severe GO failed to demonstrate a unique gene responsible for the eye disease. There are probably genetic contributions to the development of GO that do exist, but they have not yet been identified. Findings from this study suggest that environmental factors may have a more important role than genetic influences in the development of GO.

CTL 4 Genes

The presence and severity of GO has also been linked with an allele (one of the two possible genes present on a genetic locus) of the cytotoxic T lymphocyte antigen-4-gene (CTL-4). The CTL-4 gene is a co-stimulatory molecule, making it an important negative regulator of T cell activation. Researchers have discovered that the polymorphism CTL-4A/G at codon 17 of the CTL-4 gene confers susceptibility to GO. In one study published by Vaidya et al. involving 278 patients, the GG and AG genotypes were strongly associated with the development of GO. While identifying patients with this polymorphism is unlikely to become routine, this genetic link helps to explain why some people with no other risk factors (smoking, RAI, diet) may still develop severe GO.

Environmental Factors

Researchers continue to look for reasons to explain why most patients with GO merely have mild symptoms, while a smaller number of patients experience severe symptoms. One explanation is that the mild and severe forms of GO represent different disorders with different genetic profiles. Another explanation is that environmental factors shape the course of GO and determine its severity. The following environmental factors have been studied and shown to have an influence on autoimmune disease development.

Age

GO is known to develop in all age groups, although it's generally mild when it occurs in children. A recent Minnesota study showed that the age-specific incidence of GO appears to have two peak periods. In women, GO primarily develops between the ages of 40 and 44, and again between the ages of 60 and 64. In men, GO primarily develops between the ages of 45 and 49, and again between the ages of 65 and 69. This study suggests that the risk of developing GO increases with age. Lifetime exposure to environmental agents also increases with age, suggesting a role for environmental agents.

GO is generally not as severe in children as it is in adults. Studies show that children are most likely to develop lid lag and lid edema and lower lid retraction. It is very rare for children to develop symptoms that threaten vision or debilitating ocular myopathy (eye muscle disease).

Sex

While the risk of developing Graves' disease in women is nearly ten times that of men, in GO risk ratio changes. Women with thyroid disease are three times as likely as men to develop mild GO, and among people with euthyroid Graves' disease, the risks for men and women are approximately the same. The risks for developing moderate to severe GO are considerably higher in men than in women. It is thought that men do not seek medical treatment until their symptoms are more severe, when therapeutic agents are less likely to be beneficial.

Iodine

Iodine is an essential ingredient of thyroid hormone. Excess iodine is known to trigger the development of autoimmune thyroid disease. Iodine is suspected of causing increased production of TSH receptor antibodies, the antibodies responsible for causing hyperthyroidism in Graves' disease and congestive GO. In areas of adequate iodine intake, limiting iodine consumption to less than 150 mcg daily can reduce symptoms of both hyperthyroidism and GO. Iodine is an element found naturally in the soil although glacial areas are generally stripped of iodine and lacking in resources. In many parts of the world food products are subsidized with iodine to prevent iodine deficiency. Consequently, many people are at risk of ingesting excess dietary iodine. The average fast food diet contains 1,000 mcg of iodine daily. The recommended daily allowance for iodine is 75-150 mcg.

Radioiodine, which is a radioisotope of iodine created by nuclear fission, is sometimes used for the treatment of hyperthyroidism and thyroid cancer. Radioiodine either destroys or mutates cells at its path length.

Because immune system cells are stimulated by radioiodine molecules to react, titers of thyroid antibodies rise dramatically after RAI, increasing the risk for GO.

Estrogens and Endocrine Disruptors

Estrogens are a known environmental trigger for autoimmune thyroid disease. Because estrogen can influence the course in autoimmune disease, worsening symptoms, the use of estrogen supplements can contribute to symptoms in GO. Autoimmune thyroid disease, as well as GO, is also more likely to occur in the postpartum period when estrogen levels are at their highest and the immune system lapses from its pregnancy-induced suppression.

Certain chemicals, notably polychlorinated biphenyl (PCB) compounds, are also known to act as endocrine disruptors, mimicking estrogen molecules in the body although their structure is not at all similar to that of estrogen. In doing so, endocrine disruptors also increase the risk for autoimmune disease development although there have been no studies to date that show a link between endocrine disruptors and the development of GO.

Stress

Stress has profound immune system influences. Stress causes a reduction of natural killer and T suppressor lymphocytes, cells that would normally prevent autoreactive cells from multiplying and producing autoantibodies. Chronic stress is particularly devastating in that it promotes conditions favorable to autoimmune disease development

In response to stress, the endocrine glands release the stress hormones, corticotrophin releasing hormone (CRH), adrenaline, and adrenocorticotrophic hormone (ACTH). ACTH causes the adrenal gland to release cortisol. These hormones cause the body to respond in a number of different ways to help protect us against threat. The immune cells respond by becoming activated. Eventually, when the threat has passed the hormone levels return to normal and the immune system cells return to their normal activities.

Over time, when stress is chronic, cortisol levels remain elevated and immune system cells remain activated. Cortisol enlists cytokines to help, and these cytokines enable the activated immune cells to initiate an all-out autoimmune response, meaning, in the case of GO, that stress perpetuates the active disease process because thyroid autoantibody production persists. Stress is known to be the number one trigger for Graves' disease and is known to worsen symptoms in patients with GO.

Heat Shock Proteins

The immune system chemicals known as cytokines, which are released during the immune response, persist during the active phase of GO. These cytokines help to induce expression of heat shock protein (HSP) 70 and 72 on orbital fibroblast cells. These HSP molecules are important for antigen recognition and contribute to the development and progression of GO.

HSP is also expressed in patients who smoke, which is discussed further in this chapter with lifestyle factors (discussed further on), and its expression is reduced in patients who are using anti-thyroid drugs as therapy for their hyperthyroidism.

Radioiodine (I131) Therapy

Radioiodine (I131) ablative treatment for hyperthyroidism has long been suspected of contributing to the development of GO. And several large studies conducted in the last decade have definitively proven that radioiodine is capable of inducing the development of GO in patients with no signs of eye disease; and worsening GO in patients who show signs of GO before undergoing ablation.

As a protective measure, prednisone may be administered for several weeks, starting shortly before ablation. This protocol is reported to be helpful in preventing GO from occurring in the weeks following RAI. However, there are no long-term studies showing that adjunctive corticosteroids will prevent GO from eventually developing in ablated patients.

And studies of patients treated with radioiodine show that levels of TSH receptor antibodies rise significantly after RAI. In one recent study, 75 percent of patients treated with radioiodine showed increased levels of these antibodies one year after their ablations. The risk of developing GO after I 131 therapy is also higher among smokers and in patients who are allowed to become hypothyroid after ablation. Prompt institution of thyroid hormone replacement therapy reduces this risk.

Lifestyle Factors

Cigarette Smoking

Researchers at the University of Pisa in Pisa, Italy have found that cigarette smoking is a risk factor for GO. In addition, cigarette smoking decreases the efficacy of standard treatments for GO, including orbital radiation and glucocorticoid therapies.

This study included 300 patients with mild GO and an additional 150 patients with severe GO. In one phase of the study, ophthalmopathy progressed in 3 of 68 nonsmokers and in 19 of 82 smokers. GO was alleviated in 37 of 58 nonsmokers who received radioiodine ablative treatment for hyperthyroidism, along with prednisone. This suggests that although relapse of GO may occur, non-smokers initially show a much more favorable response to treatment than smokers.

While the direct effects of cigarette smoking on orbital tissue are unknown, smoking is thought to have irritating effects on orbital cells as it does on thyroid cells, and may affect immune reactions occurring in the retro-orbital space. Smoking is also known to have a negative impact on the immune system chemicals known as cytokines. And smokers have also been found to have lower serum levels of naturally occurring cytokine receptor antagonists. This is thought to be responsible for the diminished response to orbital radiotherapy seen among cigarette smokers.

Cigarette smoking is also responsible for causing increased production of soluble adhesion molecules. (Soluble adhesion molecules, immune system players that contribute to autoimmune disease development, are elevated in patients with GO.)

Furthermore, studies show that smokers have a much higher chance of developing severe GO than non-smokers. This doesn't appear to be related to the amount of cigarettes one smokes, although the association between cigarette smoking and severe GO is limited to current smokers. People with a past history of smoking who are no longer smoking have the same risk as non-smokers, suggesting that the antigens in cigarette smoke cause antigenic changes in orbital cells.

Diet

Dietary effects on autoimmunity are suspected, although such effects are controversial and further information is evolving.

Sugar and saturated fats are the primary dietary culprits in GO. Both cause immune system changes that promote inflammation. The artificial sweetener aspartame is also reported to cause immune system changes that contribute to autoimmune disease development. Other substances that tax and weaken the immune system include processed foods, refined foods, alcohol, and dairy products.

Cherries and berries, which are high in plant chemicals known as acanthocyanins, are beneficial for reducing inflammation because these chemicals act as inhibitors for cyclooxygenase and other chemicals that cause inflammation. Vegetables, especially green, yellow and orange vegetables and roots, strengthen the immune system. Chlorphyll-rich foods, such as microalgae and cereal grasses (found in health food and specialty stores), are anti-inflammatory and immune enhancing. Shiitake and reishi mushrooms are powerful immune system healers because they contain compounds known as glyconutrients (see chapter 11).

Medications

Some medications, particularly antihistamines, nasal decongestants, tranquilizers and antidepressant medications may contribute to dry eye. Recreational drugs, particularly cocaine and amphetamines, cripple the immune system and contribute to autoimmune disease. Researchers in France have reported the development of severe GO in a patient treated with interferon alpha for chronic hepatitis C. In this case, proptosis developed after three months and the active phase of the disease persisted for one year. Interferon has previously been linked to the development of autoimmune thyroid disease.

Allergens

The immune system becomes challenged when it continuously fights off allergens. In the process, it secretes high concentrations of immunoglobulin E. Immunoglobulin E is associated with more severe autoimmune disease activity. It is important to avoid known and suspected allergens, and to treat their symptoms with natural substances such as quercetin, bromelain and Vitamin C. Antihistamines and decongestants can worsen symptoms of GO.

Stress Reduction Techniques

Effectively reducing the effects of stress represents a lifestyle change that can help reduce symptoms of GO and aid in halting the active disease phase. While it is impossible and not necessarily desirable to avoid all sources of stress, it is how we deal with stress, rather than the stressor itself, that harms the immune system. The chronic effects of stress, including the stress associated with severe exercise, such as marathon racing and power weight lifting, weaken the immune system, primarily by causing the secretion of certain adrenal hormones. When they are weakened, immune system cells become ineffective. Besides allowing autoreactive cells to proliferate, weak immune system cells over-react to antigenic stimulation, setting the stage for autoimmune disease development.

Chronic stress ultimately changes the levels of immune system chemicals and cells, creating a cellular disturbance that promotes inflammation. Therapeutic programs and protocols, such as tai chi, which are designed to support and strengthen the immune system, restore these levels to their normal ranges, reducing inflammation and its associated symptoms.

Physical exercise, meditation and relaxation techniques are the key elements of stress reduction. Tai chi and yoga are effective disciplines. In some of the larger cities, yoga instructors teach programs that are specifically designed to help people with autoimmune disorders. Journal writing, social support and prayer also benefit immune system health, as do music therapy and aromatherapy.

Researchers at the University of Miami Medical School have found that daily meditation exercises that progressively release tension in muscles cause an increase in our levels of white blood cells known as T helper cells and natural killer cells. These changes are signs of an effective immune system

9
DIAGNOSIS

Because many of its symptoms are also seen in other conditions, including infection, GO may initially be difficult to diagnose. The diagnosis of Graves' ophthalmopathy is understandably simpler when patients have overt or clear-cut thyroid disease and certain symptoms characteristically seen in GO. Nevertheless, because other primary conditions can cause symptoms similar to those seen in GO, these other conditions—such as myasthenia gravis—must often be ruled out before a definitive diagnosis of GO can be made. In patients with no signs or history of thyroid disease, diagnosis is more difficult. Sophisticated ophthamological tests and imaging procedures must often be performed before a diagnosis of GO can be made.

In Thyroid Disease

In patients with overt thyroid disorders or a past history of thyroid disease, the diagnosis of Graves' ophthalmopathy is easily made when certain characteristic symptoms, such as bilateral eyelid retraction, are present. When thyroid disease cannot be established, patients are generally tested for the presence of thyroid antibodies in their blood to see if an association with autoimmune thyroid disease can be established. Thyroid antibodies are typically present in the blood of patients with autoimmune thyroid conditions, even when symptoms of thyroid disease have not yet developed.

The presence of thyroid antibodies is useful in confirming that the patient's eye symptoms are caused by GO, although GO may co-exist with other eye disorders. Thyroid antibodies include: binding, blocking and stimulating TSH (thyrotrophin) receptor antibodies; thyroid stimulating immunoglobulins (TSI); thyroid growth immunoglobulins (TGI); thyroglobulin antibodies; and thyroid peroxidase (TPO, formerly known as microsomal) antibodies. Although not all these antibodies are linked to GO, their presence in a patient with no other links to thyroid disease can establish a connection with autoimmune thyroid disease.

Diagnosing GO

Most endocrinologists examine their thyroid patients for signs of thyroid eye disease. If mild symptoms are present, the physician may wait to see if these symptoms improve with correction of the thyroid hormone levels. If the patient appears to have significant symptoms or has a strong family history of GO, the endocrinologist may refer the patient to an ophthalmologist, a physician who specializes in diagnosing and treating diseases of the eye. Some patients who show no evidence of GO and have no history of GO may want to consult with an ophthalmologist early on to obtain baseline measurements of their eyes. These can be used for comparison if the condition changes. At this initial examination, patients can also be evaluated for autoimmune changes that could interfere with vision.

With sophisticated sensitive imaging procedures, such as ultrasound, most patients with Graves' disease and a number of patients with Hashimoto's thyroiditis will show indications of GO. Yet most thyroid patients who show these signs on close examination will not go on to develop clinically significant eye disorders.

For this reason, most ophthalmologists do not complete a full diagnostic evaluation or order imaging tests on patients with Graves' disease unless symptoms and signs are present or the patient has a strong family history of GO. Even in the absence of symptoms, however, most patients with a diagnosis of Graves' disease will be examined for signs of proptosis using a Hertel exophthalmometer, which is described later in this chapter. And while the systems of classification described in chapter 4 may be included in the diagnostic work-up, they're primarily used to assess whether GO is absent, mild, moderate or severe.

Determining Severity

By assessing the signs and symptoms, taking a careful patient history, and performing certain diagnostic tests, physicians can classify GO as being mild, moderate or severe, and they can determine if the patient is in an active disease stage. Often, the symptoms that worry patients (for instance, diplopia) are considered less serious by the physician because these symptoms are likely to subside or are easy to correct. Physicians are often more concerned about slight blurring of color vision or a barely detectable field defect, since these symptoms may indicate a subtle optic neuropathy. The following tests are used to help diagnose GO, determine its severity and assess its stage and disease course.

Thyroid Tests

Thyroid Function Tests

When patients with suspected GO have no evidence or past history of thyroid disease, evidence of abnormal thyroid regulation should be sought. Patients should be tested for levels of free thyroid hormone, FT4 and FT3, and for the regulatory pituitary hormone TSH. When patients have normal thyroid hormone levels but have an abnormal TSH level, a diagnosis of subclinical thyroid disease is made. The presence of thyroid antibodies, as mentioned, helps in establishing thyroid autoimmunity.

Thyroid Antibody Titers

Certain thyroid autoantibodies are suspected of contributing to the development of GO. While GO is easily diagnosed in patients with known thyroid disease or a past history of thyroid diseases, it is more difficult to diagnose GO in patients who are euthyroid, that is, they have normal thyroid function tests. Because many of these patients may develop thyroid antibodies long before they develop signs of autoimmune thyroid disease, it is helpful to test these patients for the presence of thyroid antibodies, particularly TSH receptor antibodies. Other antibodies, including collagen stimulating immunoglobulins (CSI), have been linked to GO in early studies, but TSH receptor antibodies are the only antibodies known to have a causative relationship in GO. CSI antibodies are no longer suspected of playing a role in GO.

Recent studies show that patients with both stimulating and blocking TSH receptor antibodies are most likely to develop GO. In addition, patients with high titers of stimulating TSH receptor antibodies (also known as thyroid stimulating immunoglobulins) and no evidence of thyroid peroxidase (TPO) antibodies have a markedly increased risk of developing clinically evident ophthalmopathy.

The Eye Examination

Patients should be examined subjectively to help define the stage of their eye disease and ascertain its natural course, which is unique in each patient. Patients should be asked when they first noticed eye symptoms, and they should be asked if eye pain, lacrimation (tearing), photophobia, visual blurring and diplopia are present. Physicians should assess if the symptoms appear stable or if they have progressed. Physicians should also inquire whether the symptoms are tolerable or if they require pain relief. Patients with diplopia should be questioned to see if their diplopia is intermittent, occurring primarily in the morning, or if it is constant.

The physician will then conduct an objective examination, checking for visual acuity, papillary responses, color vision, periorbital edema, lid edema, signs of infection and lid lag. The eye exam measures certain aspects of vision and generally evaluates: visual acuity, peripheral vision, depth perception, color vision and the ability to focus on close objects.

The physician generally begins the examination by checking visual acuity in each eye, measured separately. Then he or she examines the papillary responses. When both a reduction in visual acuity and a papillary defect are present, optic neuropathy is likely and formal testing of visual fields is indicated. Certain findings noted early in the course of the examination help determine what other tests are needed.

Color Vision Testing

Acquired color vision problems can be the result of lesions of the macula, optic nerve, or visual cortex. Acquired color vision defects are generally asymmetrical in the two eyes, affecting red-green as well as yellow-blue. People with defective color vision have difficulty distinguishing certain colors. Color vision testing in each eye can help in determining optic nerve dysfunction, except in the eight percent of men who have a congenital color vision defect.

Visual Acuity Testing

Visual acuity is expressed in Snellen notation, expressed as a fraction. In the Snellen notation, the numerator indicates the test distance and the denominator denotes the distance at which the letter read by the patient subtends five minutes of arc (meaning that the letters are smaller in the next line). The Snellen eye chart is a tool widely used to measure vision. Normal vision is expressed as 20/20. An acuity of 20/60 indicates that the patient was tested at 20 feet but could only see letters that a person with normal vision could read at 60 feet.

Visual Evoked Potentials

Visual evoked potentials are an objective measurement in which patients report their response to certain stimuli. Visual evoked potentials are reportedly more sensitive in detection of optic neuropathy than visual acuity testing.

Visual Field Testing

The visual field is the total area where objects can be seen in the peripheral vision while the eye is focused on a central point. Visual field tests include: perimetry; Tangent screen exam; automated perimetry exam; Amsler grid testing; Goldmann visual field exam; and Humphrey visual field exam. In a perimetry test, patients look at a testing screen on which a computerized instrument flashes spots of light that vary in brightness. The patient presses a button whenever they see a flash. The instrument records each response. Blank holes or gaps in the field of vision are generally indications of disease.

Refraction Assessment

Refraction refers to the bending of lightwaves as they pass through your cornea and lens. A refraction assessment helps in determining what corrections are needed to provide the sharpest vision.

Slit-Lamp Examination

A slit lamp is used to examine the structures at the front of the eye under magnification. The microscope is called a slit lamp because it uses an intense line of light, a slit, to provide illumination of the cornea, iris, lens and anterior chamber. During this exam, the physician may use fluorescein dye—allowing tiny cuts, scrapes, tears, foreign material or infections of the cornea to stand out. Either fluorescein or Rose Bengal dye can be used to detect exposure keratitis.

The slit-lamp can also be used to examine the retina if dilating drops are used to widen the pupils, providing a clearer picture of the back of the eye. Using a slit-lamp or an ophthalmoscope, the doctor can diagnose abnormalities in the vitreous, retina, optic nerve and choroids.

Cover Test and Hess Screen

The cover test and Hess Screen are used to evaluate extraocular muscle alignment. These tests can be repeated, using different positions and postures, to see if abnormal head posture changes are compensating for orbital muscles that are no longer aligned properly. These manipulations can also be used to help determine which specific orbital muscle is defective. For instance, the right superior oblique muscle moves the eye down and to the left. A defect in this muscle would result in an abnormal head posture in which the chin pointed down and to the left with a tilt.

The City Hess Screen Program is a computerized tool used by ophthalmologists and orthoptists to evaluate ocular motility and determine if motility problems are constant, or change in relation to the direction of gaze. In this test, the patient wears red and blue goggles and is positioned in front of the computer monitor at an appropriate distance. With the room lights extinguished, the patient views circles and, using the mouse, moves the circles until they appear to be centered on the screen.

Fundus Examination

Fundus photography can be used to check for optic nerve damage. This method takes pictures of the optic nerve and can reveal changes years in advance of vision loss. It's an unpleasant procedure and involves the use of drops and a bright flash. The funduscopic examination is used to search for papilledema or choroidal folds, which when present in GO, are usually associated with optic neuropathy or marked orbital inflammation.

Evaluation Tools

Hertel Exophthalmometer

While other types of exophthalmometers, such as the Krahn and Luedde, are available, most ophthalmologists still use the Hertel exophthalmometer as a tool to measure proptosis. The measurement relies on an assessment of the area from the outer orbital rim (orbital wall) to the apex or highest exterior point of the cornea.

Lid Fissure Measurement

Lid fissure width and position of the lids relative to the limbus are measured using a ruler. The limbus is the marginal region of the cornea of the eye by which it is continuous with the sclera.

Lid and Conjunctival Evaluation

In this procedure, the patient is asked to close the lids lightly as in sleeping to determine if they have incomplete lid closure (lagophthalmos). Lid lag is evaluated by having the patient follow the finger of the examiner as it's moved from the up-gaze to the down-gaze position. Conjunctival injection, when it occurs, is a non-specific finding. Injection in Graves' disease is generally first noted over the insertions of the medial and lateral rectus muscles.

Ophthalmoscopy

An ophthalmoscope is an instrument used to peer through the pupil directly at the optic nerve. The optic nerve can be examined for its shape and color, and its nerve fibers can be evaluated to see if there are signs of damage related to high pressure. Damaged nerve fibers may be indicated by an asymmetrical or elongated cupped optic nerve, and by the color of the optic nerve. If damaged, it may be pale or an unhealthy pink.

Perimetry

Perimetry tests are used to check for peripheral vision, the areas of vision that extend away from the front and off to the sides. Perimetry is one of the tests used in visual field examinations.

Tonometry

Tonometry, a test widely used to diagnose glaucoma, is used to determine the pressure of the aqueous humor inside the eye. There are several methods. In the Schiotz method, the physician first anesthetizes the eye with drops, then presses very lightly against the eye with a tonometer, a small instrument used to measure pressure. In the applanation method, the physician touches a strip of orange-dyed paper to the side of the eye. The stain helps visualize changes. The physician uses a slit-lamp, which is moved forward toward the eye until the tonometer makes contact with the eye. In the non-contact approach, the physician aspirates a puff of air and measures the force needed to indent the eye.

Glycosaminoglycan (GAG) Levels

Glycosaminoglycan is a mucinous substance, primarily composed of hyaluronic acid, which contributes to congestion in GO. In congestive

GO, cells within the eye known as adipocytes produce increased levels of GAG. GAG deposits infiltrate orbital tissue, contributing to congestion. The active disease phase of GO can be evaluated by measuring levels of GAG in serum or urine, with increased levels showing an active disease process. With the introduction of sensitive tests to measure thyroid stimulating immunoglobulins (TSI), the test for GAG has largely been replaced with measurements of TSI.

Evaluation of Diplopia

Patients with diplopia are questioned to determine whether the diplopia is horizontal (two images are side by side); or vertical (two images are above each other); or oblique (two images are separated both horizontally and vertically). Patients are also questioned about the duration of the diplopia and how frequently it occurs. Patients should also be questioned about other medical conditions and medications they are using or recent trauma to the face and head.

Patients should also be evaluated to see if their diplopia is binocular, that is, it goes away when one eye is covered. Monocular diplopia, which persists with one eye covered, is rare and usually related to corneal deformity or marked astigmatism (keratoconus). The eyes should also be examined separately for visual acuity and assessed to see if looking through a pinhole improves the problem. Major differences in visual acuity suggest intraocular or refractive problems.

Patients should also be tested to see how various directions of gaze modify the diplopia. That is, is the diplopia the same when looking straight ahead or sideways. This evaluation can enhance subtle weaknesses of individual muscles that may not have shown up during testing of the range of movements. Patients should also be asked if they have symptoms of torticollis or wry neck, a painful condition that limits neck movement. Torticollis may occur over time as patients forcibly restrict their head movements to compensate for diplopia. ·

In testing for the range of movements, each eye should be examined separately, and then both eyes should be examined together. The anatomy of the extraocular muscles should be considered in determining how range of motion affects vision. The eyes are also checked to see if they adduct (turn fully inward) or abduct (turn outward). This helps in determining which eye is responsible for the diplopia. Normal contraction of the medial rectus muscle produces adduction. Contraction of the lateral rectus muscle causes abduction. The eyes are best evaluated with the eye abducted.

The inferior rectus muscle is responsible for depressing or lowering the globe; while the superior rectus muscle elevates the globe during abduction. By observing upward and downward movement, the function of the oblique muscles can be isolated. With the eyes adducted, the inferior oblique muscle elevates and the superior oblique muscle lowers the eyeball.

Tensilon Test

Intravenous injection of a short-acting anticholinesterase (10 mg/ml edrophonium chloride or Tensilon) is often included in the initial work-up for diplopia or extraocular muscle paralysis. Patients are first given a test dose of 1 mg to check for sensitivity. If there is no reaction, the remaining 9 mg are administered. A positive cholinergic response causes symptoms of salivation, lacrimation, flushing, and a brief reversal of the weakness. Excessive cholinergic stimulation can cause increased vagal tone with serious bradyarrhythmias.

Patients with other myopathies, such as GO, progressive external ophthalmoplegia or myotionia, will not respond to anticholinesterases and will show no improvement in their symptoms. The muscle weakness associated with myasthenia gravis, however, will be corrected within one minute, and the benefit will persist for several minutes.

Parks 3-Step Test

This test helps to isolate which of the four extraocular muscles responsible for vertical eye movements may be weak, thereby causing diplopia.

Forced Duction Testing

Forced duction testing is used to confirm entrapment of the inferior rectus muscle, which can contribute to strabismus.

Imaging Studies

Computed tomography, ultrasonography and magnetic resonance imaging are the primary imaging tests used to diagnose GO. Both MRI and CT reveal enlarged EOM bellies with tendon sparing, which is a diagnostic finding in GO. Imaging tests in GO also reveal maximal swelling of muscles in the mid-portion, causing: a "coke bottle" sign (meaning that the cells in the mid region of the muscle are swollen whereas the cells at the ends aren't swollen); slight uveo-scleral thickening; apical crowding; increased diameter of the optic nerve sheath; increased density of orbital fat; and anterior displacement of the lacrimal gland. Besides helping to diagnose GO and evaluate its severity, imaging tests are helpful in ruling out other causes of proptosis, such as tumors, pseudotumors and other orbital masses.

Fluorescein Angiography

Fluorescein angiography is a diagnostic test commonly used to evaluate diseases of the retina and the choroids. In this procedure, fluorescein dye is injected into an arm vein. As the dye circulates through the eye, blood vessels in the retina and choroids stand out as bright yellow. A camera takes flash pictures every few minutes, allowing assessment of damage to blood vessels.

Laser Polarimetry

Polarimetry uses laser technology to scan the eye, and doesn't require any response from the patient. This technique can measure nerve fiber thickness in the eye and reveal early signs of deterioration. Polarimetry is primarily used as a diagnostic aid for glaucoma.

Magnetic Resonance Imaging (MRI)

Magnetic resonance imaging (MRI) is a diagnostic technique that uses the magnetic properties of the hydrogen nucleus excited by radio-frequency radiation. In this procedure, a strong magnetic field is applied to the body. This excites protons in body tissues and causes them to align in an orientation particular to the magnetic field. In doing so, the protons emit a signal that is detected as induced electric currents. When the magnetic field is switched off, the protons relax to their original alignment and re-emit the gained energy.

Tissue cells that contain more hydrogen, in the form of water, can easily be distinguished from normal tissue. MRI allows for measurements of extraocular muscle thickness and the degree of proptosis, and it offers a good visualization in the critical area of the orbital axis.

Contrast-enhanced MRI has the capability of demonstrating fibrotic changes in extraocular muscles and surrounding soft tissue. T-1-weighted orbital MRI 2 or 3 mm thick images obtained in axial, coronal, and sagittal planes can be use to determine the amount of orbital fatty tissue. The amount of orbital fatty tissue is closely related to the degree of exoph-thalmos. (On T-2-1 scans, for example, enlarged eye muscles demonstrate a high signal intensity.)

Gadolinium contrast dye can be given intravenously to help enhance imaging. After gadolinium administration, MRI can distinguish between muscles that are swollen due to fatty degeneration, fibrosis, or edema. In GO, the amount of orbital fatty tissue may be much greater than that of extraocular muscle.

High resolution MRI is also able to depict all of the major blood vessels and cranial nerves of the orbit as well as the major septa of the orbital connective tissue system. MRI offers the advantage of not exposing the lens to radiation. However, the procedure takes longer and it is generally more expensive than CT.

STIR MRI

Serial short tau inversion recovery (STIR) sequence magnetic resonance imaging (MRI) scans are another useful tool for measuring inflammatory activity in extraocular muscles. The signal intensity ratio of the most inflamed extraocular muscle correlates well with the clinical activity score (CAS) of Mourits, meaning that the signal intensity ratio is higher in patients with worse or progressive symptoms, showing that the signal intensity can be used to diagnose the active phase of GO.

Ocreotide Scintigraphy

In active GO, Octreoscan imaging studies using the somatostatin analog 1111 n-ocreotide (which is a chemical similar in structure to one of the body's neurohormones, known as somatostatin), shows a high orbital uptake. Ocreotide is able to bind to the cell membrane of activated lymphocytes expressing somatostatin receptors, and a significant tracer accumulation in the retrobulbar space is seen in active GO.

In this procedure, ocreotide uptake is measured at 4 and 24 hours following the injection of approximately 3 mCi of 111 Indium-DTPA-Ocreotide with a neuro-SPECT camera. Counts are measure in fixed regions of the orbital area. Using the orbital/occipital ratio of the four-hour scan, patients can be evaluated for disease activity.

Orbital Gallium 67 Scintigraphy

In this procedure, orbital gallium 67 citrate is administered intravenously, and the amount of gallium taken up by orbital cells is measured after 48 hours using scintigraphy. Single photon emission computed (SPECT) images are obtained using a gamma camera. Orbital uptake of gallium 67 is significantly increased in the active phase of GO. In studies using this protocol, patients treated with immunosuppressant therapy were retested six months later at which time the orbital uptake of gallium 67 was significantly decreased.

Orbital Computed Tomography (CT) Scans

Computed tomography is a diagnostic imaging technique used to determine structural anatomy. Currently, it's the most valuable technique for delineating the shape, locations, extent and character of orbital lesions. It is particularly helpful in diagnosing GO, determining its severity, and excluding other causes of proptosis. CT may be used to estimate the volume of extraocular muscle and retro-ocular fat tissue. In doing so, CT allows measurements of extraocular thickness and the degree of proptosis; and it offers good visualization in the critical area of the orbital axis.

Computed tomography relies on the same principles as x-rays and measures changes in orbital anatomy based on differences in the ability of tissue to absorb x-rays. Computed tomography, with axial and coronal views, is the preferred study because this technique offers good resolution of bony detail and its cost is lower. Coronal CT scanning is especially useful in evaluating orbital floor fractures and extraocular muscle size.

Improved technologies allowing for higher resolution images and multiplanar imaging have made CT a valuable tool. In orbital imaging, iodinated contrast material is rarely used because it delays future radioiodine treatment. In addition, because iodine is a known trigger for autoimmune thyroid disease, it can exacerbate symptoms of thyrotoxicosis.

Radiolabeled somatostatin analogues such as ocreotide are taken up by orbital tissue in patients with active GO. The extent of uptake may correlate with clinical responsiveness to immunosuppressive or somatostatin-analogue (ocreotide) therapy. Patients in the active phase of GO who are responding positively to steroid therapy or external beam radiation, will have lower ocreotide uptakes than that seen on their initial diagnostic tests.

Because CT is used to measure the posterior corneal surface, this technique cannot be used to compare measurements of proptosis taken by exophthalmometry. Exophthalmometry techniques measure the anterior corneal surface, and the anterior corneal surface can normally exceed the posterior surface, which is measured using CT, by as much as 5 mm. In evaluating patients to see if there's a worsening of their condition or a favorable response to therapy, the same method should be used consistently.

Single Photon/Positron Emission Computed Tomography (SPECT)

SPECT is an imaging technique capable of assessing function in relative or absolute terms. In SPECT, patients receive injections of compounds, such as glucose, that are normally used by orbital cells, to measure cellular activity or blood flow in specific tissues.

Ultrasonography

Ultrasonography (ultrasound) is a non-invasive imaging technique based on the principle that body tissues have a property called "acoustic impedance." Sound waves entering tissue can be either transmitted through the tissue or reflected, depending on their density. Advantages of ultrasound include its ease of use, lack of ionizing radiation, excellent tissue differentiation and cost effectiveness. For these reasons, ultrasound is often used before CT or MRI as a first-line study.

A-mode ultrasonography is an excellent tool for diagnosing GO. It is considered a better tool for detecting subtle changes in soft orbital tissue and for differentiating extraocular muscles and optic nerve lesions than routine ultrasound. Ultrasound, including colour Doppler ultrasonography, is excellent for diagnosing vascular lesions and for assessing orbital circulation.

However, for assessing disease activity or response, objective measurements are more reliable than ultrasonography. In addition, ultrasound is inferior to CT and MRI for depicting the bony wall, orbital apex, adjacent sinuses and intracranial compartments. Ultrasound also has the disadvantage of not being able to examine both eyes simultaneously.

T2 Relaxation Time at MRI

Relaxation time can be measured with T-weighted MRI, with a prolonged T2 relaxation time indicative of active GO.

Eye Muscle Reflectivity (EMR)

Eye muscle reflectivity can also be used to indicate disease progression. EMR can be measured by A-mode ultrasonography. An EMR of 40 percent or less is indicative of active GO.

Signs and Symptoms

A diagnostic work-up for Graves' ophthalmopathy also includes an assessment of the many signs and symptoms that accompany GO. These were described in chapter 2. Because symptoms in GO may wax and wane, patients should be asked for a complete medical history, including a history of past or intermittent signs and symptoms. This will help their physicians determine if their disease course is particularly progressive. Patients should also be asked for a list of current medications since many common medications, including antihistamines, will affect symptoms in GO.

Evaluating Intraocular Pressure

When patients with GO develop increased intraocular pressure, it is important to determine the cause. Some patients with GO simultaneously develop glaucoma, which may require different treatment. Intraocular pressure elevations in GO may also be related to impaired venous circulation, compression by infiltrative muscles, and long-term corticosteroid use. Tests for visual acuity and perimetry can be used to help differentiate glaucoma from pressure changes related to GO, since patients with glaucoma show distinct defects in perimetry tests.

Other Causes of Ophthalmopathy

When a diagnosis of thyroid disease is uncertain, patients need to be evaluated carefully to look for other causes of ophthalmopathy.

Other conditions that cause proptosis include:

- myopia;
- certain brain lesions;
- cirrhosis; congenital anomalies; medications (lithium, steroids, cold pills, diet medications);
- contralateral ptosis;
- illusory ptosis of the opposite eyelid;
- carotid cavernous fistula; infection;
- inflammation; hydrocephalus;
- hypokalemic periodic paralysis;
- Cushing's syndrome;

- chronic obstructive lung disease;
- uremia;
- myasthenia gravis; and
- nervous system lesions.

Bilateral proptosis may be caused by:

- shallow orbits (Crouzon's disease);
- large globes (characteristic of severe myopia); and
- retro-ocular fat accumulation (in Cushing's syndrome and obesity).

Bilateral proptosis may also occur in:

- lithium therapy;
- Wegener's granulomatosis;
- lymphoma;
- arteriovenous malformations;
- idiopathic inflammatory pseudotumors;
- metastatic neuroblastoma; and
- metastatic tumors.

(Bilateral proptosis alone, while common in GO, is not diagnostic for GO.)

Chronic unilateral proptosis may occur in:

- pseudotumors;
- lymphoma;
- cavernous hemangioma;
- lacrimal gland tumor; peripheral nerve tumor; meningioma; mucocele;
- metastatic tumors; and
- secondary tumors.

Ultrasound or computed tomography can easily differentiate between these disorders because of its ability to visualize tissue masses.

Patients with GO can also have concurrent medical conditions that may contribute to ocular symptoms. These other conditions need to be ruled out before starting treatment for GO. Patients with GO can develop glaucoma. When this occurs, the infiltrated muscles can cause globe compression. Patients with Graves' disease can rarely have myasthenia gravis, an autoimmune disorder with eye symptoms similar to those seen in GO.

EMO Syndrome

EMO is a rare complication of Graves' disease in which patients exhibit exophthalmos, pretibial myxedema and osteoarthropathy (condition of soft tissue swelling in fingers and toes). The presence of pretibial myxedema, which causes waxy lesions and mottled, swollen skin primarily in the lower legs and feet, and osteoarthropathy in a patient with proptosis, helps to confirm that the eye condition is related to autoimmune thyroid disease. The osteoarthropathy may cause the fingers to appear clubbed and the skin of both legs may have red-brown waxy plaques.

Pseudotumor Cerebri

Pseudotumor cerebri is a condition in which high pressure inside the head results in swelling of the optic disc, which can result in headache and problems with vision. Patients with pseudotumor cerebri have optic disc swelling but no evidence of tumor. In pseudotumor cerebri, cerebrospinal fluid—the fluid that bathes the brain and spinal cord—is blocked from flowing normally. This causes the elevated pressure. The pressure is transmitted to the back of the eye via the optic nerve sheath (which surrounds each of the optic nerves). This produces the disc swelling (papilledema).

It is not clear exactly what causes the blocked outflow of cerebrospinal fluid. It occurs most often in young, overweight women, suggesting a hormonal influence. Some medications, particularly antibiotics and high doses of Vitamin A, may also lead to increased intracranial (within the brain) pressure.

Symptoms in pseudotumor cerebri include visual loss and a headache that frequently occurs in the back of the head. Unlike migraine, the headache associated with this condition may wake the patient up at night. The optic nerve swelling may eventually lead to loss of vision seen as dimming, blurring or graying of vision. Diagnosis can be confirmed by a normal MRI and elevated cerebrospinal fluid pressure (as measured during a spinal tap).

Optic Neuritis

Optic neuritis is an autoimmune condition in which the immune system attacks the myelin coating that covers the optic nerve. Viruses are suspected of triggering the autoimmune response in the autoimmune disorder known as optic neuritis. Optic neuritis causes a sudden decrease in vision, blurred vision, or dark vision.

Myasthenia Gravis

The autoimmune disorder myasthenia gravis (MG) poses diagnostic difficulties because, besides causing similar symptoms to those seen in GO, patients may have both GO and MG simultaneously. MG, which interferes with nerve conduction in skeletal muscles, causes muscle weakness in various organs of the body.

In MG, weakened levator muscles cause eyelid drooping. And weakened extraocular muscles cause diplopia. In contrast, when GO causes upper eyelid retraction or "lateral lid flare," it is typically the result of eyelid inflammation and fibrosis of the lateral levator horn, a small projection extending from the lateral levator muscle.

Patients suspected of having MG should have Tensilon tests, described earlier in this chapter, or blood tests to check for acetylcholine receptor antibodies. Acetylcholine receptor antibodies, which are autoantibodies responsible for the impaired innervation of muscle in MG, are generally positive in patients with myasthenia gravis, although a small number of patients with Graves' disease may also have positive acetylcholine receptor antibody titers. However, the titers of acetylcholine receptor antibodies in patients with Graves' disease are much lower than those seen in patients with MG.

10

CONVENTIONAL TREATMENT OPTIONS

There are various treatments used to alleviate symptoms in patients with GO. One of the simplest treatments involves correcting abnormal thyroid hormone levels. Most people with GO notice improvement in their eye symptoms when their thyroid hormone levels are corrected and brought into the normal range. And some people, particularly those with dry eye symptoms, notice a reduction in symptoms when they eliminate risk factors such as smoking.

In some instances, correcting thyroid hormone levels or avoiding smoking are the only treatment measures needed for patients with GO. Patients with mild GO generally do not require specific or aggressive treatment because this condition tends to improve spontaneously.

Other patients, especially those who are sensitive to light or experience dryness, may not notice improvement until they employ local protective measures, such as sunglasses or the use of ophthalmic moisture drops. (Local protective measures are described later in this chapter.) Most patients with GO can be successfully treated with local protective measures and reassurance from an expert in the field that their condition is self-limited.

Who Needs Aggressive Treatment?

Most patients with GO do not require aggressive treatment because their conditions are generally mild and self-limited. However, when the signs and symptoms of thyroid related eye disease are moderate to severe, patients may require aggressive treatment measures. Certain specific conditions that accompany GO may also indicate that therapy is needed.

Patients who are candidates for therapy include those with the following conditions:

- sight threatening ophthalmopathy;
- corneal perforation risk;
- advanced soft-tissue inflammation;
- ophthalmoplegia;
- history of globe subluxation (dislocation);
- moderate to severe proptosis;
- optic neuropathy or optic nerve compression risk; and
- distressing appearance.

Although symptoms such as extraocular muscle dysfunction may not threaten vision, the resulting diplopia may interfere with daily activities sufficiently to also require aggressive intervention, especially if it causes constant discomfort. Diplopia that requires an abnormal head position to correct it is also an indication for aggressive treatment. A worsening in proptosis or other symptoms over time, which suggests a rapidly progressive disease, is another indication for aggressive treatment.

The optimal approach to treating severe GO lies in choosing appropriate treatment modalities at the right time and in the correct sequence. The goals of treatment are to prevent visual loss, improve function and appearance, and to provide counseling and psychological support. In most cases, the patient's endocrinologist and ophthalmologist or neuro-ophthalmologist work together to manage the patient's condition.

Deciding on Treatment

When treatment for GO is indicated, there is no general consensus as to what type of treatment is best, or in which order therapy should be instituted. However, there are certainly rules and guidelines that most ophthalmologists are in agreement on. In most cases, endocrinologists can manage symptoms by controlling thyroid hormone levels and reducing symptoms of hyperthyroidism while ensuring that hypothyroidism does not develop. Anti-thyroid drugs such as methimazole (Tapazole) or propylthiouracil (PTU) help in that they block thyroid hormone synthesis and mildly suppress the immune system. The beta adrenergic blocking agent or beta blocker propranolol is effective in decreasing hypermetabolic symptoms related to excess thyroid hormone. For symptoms of congestive infiltration, or to obtain baseline eye measurements, patients may want to consult an ophthalmologist.

Because treatment undertaken at the wrong time or in the wrong sequence is ineffective, it is important to find an ophthalmologist or neuro-ophthalmologist experienced in treating GO. Systemic steroids, immunosuppressive agents and orbital radiotherapy can be used for the management of severe symptoms, but they are only effective during the active disease phase. Today, surgical orbital decompression procedures are used as a last resort.

Because GO is unique to each patient, the type of treatment used depends on the patient's particular symptoms and signs; the phase of the disease; the treatment used to regulate the thyroid disorder; the doctor's experience using various therapies; and any complicating factors, such as co-existing conditions. For instance, both glucocorticoid therapy and external beam radiation treatment (XRT) may be contraindicated in patients with diabetes because they are already at risk for developing retinopathy, which may occur as a side effect of these therapies.

Treatment Goals

For patients with the congestive, infiltrative form of GO, treatment has two goals: reducing the swollen soft tissues or expanding the orbital volume. High dose corticosteroids, other immunosuppressant (chemotherapeutic) agents, external beam radiotherapy and surgical decompression are the treatments most often employed.

The stage of the ophthalmopathy, that is, the active or the plateau phase, must be taken into consideration when evaluating available therapies. Treatment is usually initiated in the active or ascendant disease phase in an effort to protect vision and reduce symptoms. While GO is active, non-surgical therapies such as steroids, immunosuppressants or external beam radiation are usually used because they are directed at the lymphocytes perpetuating the autoimmune process. Patients with active disease generally show both symptoms and signs of active inflammation. The clinical activity score of Mourits, levels of TSH receptor antibodies, and various imaging techniques can be used to determine or confirm that the disease is in the active stage.

During the plateau phase when symptoms appear to have stabilized, treatment is generally not effective. This is because treatment is generally directed at autoreactive lymphocytes in the orbital area, and during the plateau phase, the number of autoreactive lymphocytes in the area is greatly reduced.

In the late phase, when the disease is no longer active, treatments are generally rehabilitative or corrective—intended to relieve pain, provide better coverage of the globe, correct diplopia, and improve appearance. (For more information on the various disease stages in GO see chapters 4 and 8.)

In general, surgery is withheld until the hot or active phase of the eye disorder has stabilized. However, when vision-threatening complications occur, treatment is usually more aggressive, and it may be necessary to perform surgery before stabilization occurs, particularly if fibrosis has developed

Two Rules of Treatment

While there is no optimal treatment for all patients with GO, there are two rules of treatment that ophthalmologists agree upon:

1. If a patient is losing vision from a compressive optic neuropathy despite corticosteroid treatment and/or irradiation, the patient should undergo surgical decompression.

2. The order of surgical treatment is as important as the treatment itself. In surgical rehabilitation, orbital decompression should be performed first because ocular motility can be affected by the decompression. Furthermore, strabismus surgery should precede eyelid repair because the globe position must be stable in order to place the eyelid in the correct position, and muscle surgery can change the eyelid position. Thus, orbital decompression, if required, should precede strabismus repair, which, in turn, should precede eyelid repair.

Comparing Treatment Options

Deciding on what treatment to use when vision is not threatened is occasionally left up to the patient after being presented with a number of options. The following review of long-term studies evaluating treatment options and the description of available treatment options is intended to help with the decision-making process.

Long Term Studies

The natural course and effects of different treatment protocols for GO have been poorly documented in the medical literature. For this reason, several researchers have conducted studies evaluating the treatment response of previously treated patients.

In one Swiss study of 196 patients with hyperthyroidism described by Noth, 81 were found to have signs and symptoms of GO. Only the patients with moderate to severe signs and symptoms were treated, while the others were evaluated for a period of time ranging from 1.0 to 8.9 years. The results of this study were comparable to similar studies, and showed that most patients with GO improve spontaneously. Only a small number of patients in this study had severe ocular signs and symptoms. Researchers concluded that treatment of complex cases of GO necessitates cooperation between endocrinologists, ophthalmologists, radiotherapists, and surgeons specializing in orbital procedures.

In his intensive study of treatment options, Dr. Luigi Bartalena emphasizes that glucocorticoids and irradiation (medical therapies) may help intervene directly in the disease process because of their effects on immune system cells. Surgical decompression is not intended to address the etiology or causes of GO. Rather, it is specifically intended to reduce the mechanical effects of GO.

Bartalena also emphasizes that choosing medical or surgical treatment first doesn't mean that the patient won't later require the other form of therapy. He also notes that geographical location plays a role in the type of therapy recommended. Among European endocrinologists, glucocorticoid therapy is most often recommended for GO; whereas at Mayo Clinic—where physicians have more experience with surgery—surgery is more likely to be recommended as an initial treatment.

Early studies evaluating treatment options primarily focused on measurements of proptosis, which, Bartalena warns, can be misleading. He recommends evaluating more relevant measures, including lid fissure width, range of extraocular motion on perimeter, volume of extraocular muscles and volume of retrobulbar tissue. Other parameters helpful in evaluating treatment response include dry eye and vision signs and symptoms.

Non-Surgical Treatment Options

Non-surgical treatment options, such as protective measures, glucocorticoids, other immunosuppresant medications, and orbital radiation are all reported to reduce symptoms in about two-thirds of patients. When a combination of non-surgical treatments is used, a higher percentage of patients report experiencing improvement.

Thyroid Eye Disease

Plasmapharesis (a medical procedure described later in this chapter) effectively removes circulating antibodies and other immune system chemicals that perpetuate the disease process. Diuretics are occasionally used to reduce the fluid retention characteristically seen in periorbital edema. However, their use is not generally recommended because of the potential these drugs have for depleting minerals, particularly potassium and magnesium.

Correcting Thyroid Hormone Levels

One of the simplest non-surgical options involves correcting thyroid hormone levels. Correcting thyroid hormone levels reduces symptoms directly related to excess or deficient thyroid hormone. The stare and lid retraction associated with thyroxine-induced sensitization of Mueller's muscle to circulating catecholamines (epinephrine and norepinephrine) often improve after resolution of the hyperthyroid state. However, symptoms related to the congestive, infiltrative type of GO will generally persist until the active disease phase has subsided even when thyroid hormone levels have been corrected.

Protective Measures

Localized protective measures include: avoiding winds and fan; using visors; wearing dark or tinted glasses; applying cool compresses; elevating the head of the bed at night; applying eye drops and gels; protective eye patches; and taping the eyes shut at night. Moisture shields that can be attached to the temples or spectacles help to preserve tears and retard tear evaporation.

Dark glasses and visors help protect the cornea against the sun, wind, and airbone particle irritants that promote dryness. In addition, they help prevent corneal drying and exposure keratopathy. Dark glasses and visors also help in controlling symptoms of photophobia (light sensitivity). Elevating the head of the bed at night is an effective treatment for reducing symptoms of periorbital edema.

Fluid Intake

Patients with GO often mistakenly assume that restricting fluids will improve symptoms of puffiness and dry eye. On the contrary, fluid restriction leads to increased edema because in dehydration the body retains fluids. Patients with GO should be reminded to drink adequate fluids to prevent dehydration.

Lubricants & Tear Supplements

Artificial tears, which lubricate the eye, are the principal treatment for dry eye. Tear supplements consisting of 0.3-0.75 percent methylcellulose used as eyedrops or as topical ointments (suggested products listed below), help to restore moisture and prevent foreign-body sensations and feelings of grittiness. Topical sterile ointments and lubricants can be applied in a heavy layer before taping the eyes shut at night. Alternately, after applying ointment, the eyes can be covered with a layer of cellophane (Saran Wrap) and taped, or swimming goggles may be worn. Both of these techniques help the eyes retain moisture.

Nocturnal taping also helps reduce symptoms of lid lag. However, patients with proptosis severe enough to require nocturnal taping should be under the care of an ophthalmologist so that they can be checked for exposure keratopathy or other complications. Increased corneal exposure can lead to corneal abrasions.

For nocturnal taping, apply a thick layer of tear supplement over the eye. Keeping the eye shut squeeze the cheek below the affected eye, moving it upward, and place mild Millipore tape vertically from the eyebrow down to the cheek. This technique allows for the cheek to assist in keeping the eye shut. Additional pieces of tape can then be placed horizontally, near the top and bottom of the vertical tape.

Note: according to Dr. Charles Soparkar, eye drops intended to reduce eye redness should never be used in GO. The ingredients in these products may exacerbate symptoms and contribute to blindness.

Suggested Lubricating Ointments
- LacriLube™
- Refresh PM™
- Tears Renewed™
- DuoLube®

Suggested Artificial Tears
- Celluvisc™
- Tears Naturale™
- Moisture Drops®
- Hypo Tears™
- Genteal™

Other Remedies for Dry Eye

Avoiding medications that contribute to dryness, particularly antihistamines, nasal decongestants, tranquilizers and antidepressants, will benefit patients with dry eye symptoms. Humidifiers are also helpful in that they increase the amount of moisture in the air. In cases of severe dry eye, ophthalmologists may insert plugs that cause temporary or permanent closure of the tear drain (small openings at the inner corner of the eyelids where tears drain from the eye). More self-care suggestions can be found in chapter 11.

Prisms

Prism lenses are generally used to correct minor degrees of diplopia. Prisms can be ground into lenses or applied to normal glasses using Fresnel prisms. Both techniques are effective, although Fresnel prisms are less expensive and are often used initially to see if prism therapy is sufficient to correct symptoms. Fresnel prisms always knock down vision by 1-3 lines, meaning that while the diplopia is corrected, vision is further reduced.

Patching and Stick-On Occlusive Lenses

While these are not used as often, patients may be prescribed eye patches or occlusive lenses to temporarily correct symptoms of diplopia.

Beta Adrenergic Blocking Agents

Eye drops containing beta adrenergic blocking agents, such as timolol, are also effective in reducing symptoms of increased intraocular pressure. Increased intraocular pressure may occur in GO, or it may occur as co-existing glaucoma. It is important that patients with increased intraocular pressure be evaluated carefully and examined for glaucoma.

Corticosteroids (Glucocorticoids)

Corticosteroids are effective anti-inflammatory and immunosuppressive agents, showing a favorable response in about two-thirds of patients. Glucocorticoids have been a mainstay of treatment for more than 40 years. Although this class of drugs includes a number of different compounds, prednisone is the corticosteroid most often used for GO.

Besides inhibiting the immune response, corticosteroids may also directly inhibit the synthesis of glycosaminoglycan and its release from orbital fibroblasts. Corticosteroids reduce swelling and they relieve pain, injection, and conjunctival edema, particularly that associated with soft tissue inflammation and compressive optic neuropathy. Consequently, glucocorticoids can improve proptosis, although symptoms of active inflammation may be exacerbated after treatment is withdrawn if the immune process in GO is still active.

Predicting who will respond

Glucocorticoid therapy is reported to be most effective in patients who have disease of shorter duration. However, patients with long-standing disease may also experience improvement. Other factors that predict a favorable response include: active inflammation, a high degree of signal on MRI, and uptake of radiolabeled ocreotide by retro-orbital tissues.

Dosage

Glucocorticoids may be administered orally, locally through injections or intravenously. High doses of oral prednisone (1–2 mg/kg of body weight, up to 80 mg daily) are generally used for the treatment of optic neuropathy. Usually, therapy is initiated with 60–80 mg prescribed daily for 2–4 weeks, followed by 2.5–10 mg prescribed daily for 2–4 weeks if tolerated well. At this dose, patients can expect relatively rapid improvement in visual acuity over the course of several days. Regression of chemosis and related symptoms occurs within 48 hours.

Continued improvement occurs over weeks if the dose is maintained. After several weeks, the dose is gradually reduced, with a low dose given every other day to reduce the chance of side effects. Extraocular muscle improvement, if it occurs at all, may require several weeks of therapy.

Depot subconjunctival or retro-bulbar (directly into the orbital area) injections of a glucocorticoid, usually methylprednisone, are occasionally used to limit the systemic effects of orally administered glucocorticoids. However, the associated risk and discomfort limit the usefulness of this approach.

Intravenous pulse therapy has also been used in an attempt to reduce the effects of chronic oral therapy. Methylprednisolone acetate is generally administered in doses of 0.5–1.0 gm at different intervals, with a cumulative dose of 1–21 gm. Favorable effects have been observed on inflammatory signs and optic nerve involvement. However, according to a review of the medical literature, the effects on extraocular muscle involvement and proptosis haven't been as impressive. Patients with severe GO and high titers of TSH receptor antibodies are also reported to show more improvement than patients with mild symptoms. However, in between intravenous doses, patients have generally been given oral corticosteroids, making it difficult to compare the effects of intravenous and oral agents. There are also no well-controlled studies comparing routes of drug administration.

The simultaneous administration of glucocorticoid-sparing immunosuppressant drugs such as cyclosporine A is another option used in an attempt to reduce the side effects of glucocorticoid steroids.

Side Effects

Side effects of glucocorticoid steroids include: hypertension; insomnia; weight gain; bone loss; depression; psychosis; peptic ulcer; hirsutism (facial hair); infections; cataract; glucose intolerance; and incomplete disease reversal in some cases. The precise prevalence of side effects is uncertain. In one study, major side effects included severe depression and infection and moderate side effects included hypertension, severe heartburn, hirsutism (increased facial hair), behavioral changes, and weight gain. Because corticosteroids have so many undesirable effects, other immunosuppressant drugs are often administered simultaneously so that a smaller amount of corticosteroids can be used. When immunosuppressant drugs are prescribed in this way, they are known as glucocorticoid-sparing immunosuppressive agents.

Immunosuppressants

Other immunosuppressive drugs are occasionally used in GO—both alone and in conjunction with glucocorticoids—although the experience is limited to a small series of patients treated in uncontrolled clinical trials. The agents most commonly used include: cyclosporine A; azathioprine; cyclophosphamide; pentoxyfylline; ocreotide; ciamexone; and intravenous immunoglobulins (although in controlled trials, ciamexone and cyclophosphamide showed little benefits).

Cyclosporine A

Cyclosporine A is reported to inhibit the proliferation of helper T cells and the production of immune system chemicals known as cytokines, both of which contribute to the development of GO. Cyclosporine A also inhibits the production of autoantibodies by B cells. In studies, the administration of Cyclosporine A with glucocorticosteroids proved to be more efficacious than the use of Cyclosporine A alone. In one study, 60 percent of patients who showed no response to either therapy responded to combined therapy.

However, Cyclosporine A is very expensive and it has its own potential for side effects, including diplopia, hypertension and infection. Studies also show benefits occur most often in the early stages of the immune response, and are most likely to cause improvement in patients with a sudden onset of symptoms.

Ocreotide

The chemical ocreotide is similar to the natural hormone somatostatin. Patients who have been tested and found to have somatostatin receptors in the eye muscles that show localization of nuclear isotopes with Ocreotide III scanning have experienced improvement in clinical trials using 300 mcg of ocreotide daily. However, side effects associated with this therapy make it prohibitive for most patients.

In one early trial, a small group of patients treated with ocreotide for 3 months experienced amelioration of soft-tissue changes or improvement in extraocular muscle function. In a second trial, 7 of 12 patients with active GO experienced improvement in eye index score after 3 months of ocreotide therapy. Results of these and other studies suggest that positive octreoscans might be used as a diagnostic tool for GO and a means to evaluate response to treatment.

Ocreotide is very expensive and has a short half-life. Its use requires repeated injections during the day, although some longer- acting preparations such as lanreotide have been recently introduced and the effects of ocreotide and lanreotide are reported to be comparable. While results appear promising, additional controlled studies are required before sound conclusions regarding the efficacy of these compounds can be established.

Colchicine

The anti-inflammatory agent colchicine has been studied for its effects on GO, and the results have been favorable. More controlled studies are needed before its use can be deemed efficacious. In studies, colchicine has been found to decrease the expression of certain cytokine receptors and inhibit immunoglobulin secretion, effectively reducing levels of autoantibodies.

Pentoxyfylline

Pentoxyfylline is one of the newer immunosuppressive drugs used to treat symptoms of GO. In one small study, pentoxyfylline reduced soft-tissue inflammation, but not proptosis or ophthalmoplegia. In test tube studies, these changes were associated with decreased production of GAG rather than changes to cytokines or lymphocytes.

Methotrexate

The chemotherapeutic agent methotrexate has also been successfully used for the treatment of GO. Researchers at Casey Eye Institute in Portland used methotrexate as a corticosteroid sparing agent for up to 47 months in patients with a variety of orbital inflammatory diseases, including GO.

Intravenous Immunoglobulins (IVIGs)

High dose IVIGs have been successfully used in a number of different autoimmune diseases. Intravenously administered immunoglobulin solutions work by blocking the production of new antibodies, inhibiting or modulating immune system chemicals known as cytokines; and by dissolving immune complexes (composed of antigens and antibodies; these complexes are particularly destructive to the kidneys of patients with systemic lupus). IVIG preparations also include immunosuppressive cytokines.

Results of clinical trials in GO have been conflicting with three studies showing benefits and another study showing no significant changes. Adverse effects were lower than those seen in patients using glucocorticoid steroids. Side effects are similar to those of other human derived blood products. Furthermore, because IVIGs are derived from human blood donors, availability depends on a sufficient donor population.

Plasmapheresis

In plasmapheresis, phlebotomy is performed and one unit of blood is withdrawn. The cells are removed from the plasma and transfused back into the patient. Thus, the immunoglobulins and immune complexes responsible for causing symptoms in GO are removed since they are exclusively found in plasma, which is the liquid fraction of blood. The efficacy of plasmapheresis has been examined in several small trials, but results have been conflicting. Benefits occur most often in patients with rapidly progressive forms of GO. Patients with long-standing symptoms who are most likely to have fibrosis showed little or no improvement.

In one trial, patients showed no significant improvement in proptosis, extraocular muscle dysfunction, visual acuity, visual fields, intraocular pressure or appearance of the extraocular muscles when examined with ultrasonography or computed tomography (CT) imaging. In another study, plasmapheresis followed by immunosuppressant therapy resulted in significant improvement in soft-tissue inflammation, proptosis, intraocular pressure, and extraocular muscle function.

In this procedure, patients are generally subjected to 4 plasmapheresis sessions over a period of 5–8 days followed by combined immunosuppressive therapy for 3–6 months. Because of the conflicting responses reported in studies, plasmapheresis is generally reserved for patients who have failed to respond to other forms of therapy.

Diuretics

Diuretics, such as hydrochlorothiazide in doses of 25 mg twice daily, are used to help reduce orbital fluid retention. Because diuretics can promote mineral loss, patients on diuretics should be regularly tested for potassium, magnesium and calcium, and prescribed supplements if these levels become too low.

Thyroid Ablation

Thyroid surgery is occasionally used to treat GO in an attempt to remove thyroid antigens. The rationale behind this is that the removal of thyroid antigens, which are also expressed by orbital fibroblast cells, can reduce the immune response. However, total thyroid ablation using both thyroidectomy and high doses of I 131 has not proven successful. In one large retrospective study, GO developed in 7 percent of patients following thyroidectomy, and in patients with preexisting GO, 19 percent of patients reported a progression of symptoms after surgery.

Anti-Thyroid Drugs

The anti-thyroid drugs (ATDs) methimazole and propylthiouracil are frequently prescribed for hyperthyroid patients. ATDs inhibit the production of thyroid hormone, relieving symptoms related to thyroid excess in hyperthyroid patients. ATDs also mildly suppress the immune system, and their beneficial role in the treatment of GO has been evaluated in several studies. Overall, the majority of patients with mild to moderate symptoms of GO experience an improvement in their condition while they are taking anti-thyroid drugs.

When anti-thyroid drugs are successful in eliciting remission (defined by a reduction of thyroid stimulating immunoglobulins into the normal range), symptoms of GO generally resolve permanently. However, it's important that patients using ATDs not be made hypothyroid because eye symptoms can worsen. Patients using ATDs need to have their levels of FT4 and FT3 measured every four to six weeks, and they should be instructed to be on the alert for symptoms of hypothyroidism.

Patients using ATDs who achieve remission from Graves' disease may occasionally relapse and experience a return of hyperthyroidism, especially if they are not weaned slowly from ATDs, their levels of stimulating TSH receptor antibodies are still elevated, or they are exposed to certain environmental triggers (including stress, increased estrogens, cigarette smoke and excess iodine). When this happens, symptoms of GO related to excess thyroid hormone may also return. A relapse or flare of autoimmune GO symptoms may also rarely occur after the initial disorder.

Orbital Radiotherapy (Irradiation)

External beam orbital irradiation, which has been used as a treatment for GO for more than 60 years, is generally administered in a dose of 20 Gy given in 10 fractions over two weeks. Following this protocol, irradiation may help reduce the soft tissue signs of GO, and ameliorate compressive optic neuropathy. Most treatment centers utilize linear accelerators delivering 4–6 megavolts angled posteriorly to avoid irradiating the contralateral lens. There have also been reports of success administering smaller doses over a longer period of time, although there have been no advantages reported with using doses higher than 20 Gy.

Originally, radiotherapy was directed to the hypothalamus and the pituitary because it was thought that GO was of pituitary or hypothalamic origin. In later years, radiotherapy was directed to orbital tissue, the true target of the pathological process in GO. Initially, there may be a temporary exacerbation or worsening of eye symptoms, but this is unlikely to occur if glucocorticoids are administered simultaneously.

Radiotherapy is reported to be not as successful as corticosteroids in reducing proptosis or managing diplopia, and improvement is not always noticeable until some time after therapy is completed (although improvement has been noted as early as one to four weeks after the completion of therapy).

Orbital irradiation presumably works by killing retrobulbar lymphocytes and inducing their cell death (apoptosis). These lymphocytes have been found to be very sensitive to radiation. Because lymphocytes are responsible for producing the antibodies that cause congestive GO, reducing their numbers causes an eventual reduction in congestive GO. Similar to the use of corticosteroid therapy, it's difficult to tell who will benefit, and about one-third of treated patients experience no benefits, and improvement in those who do respond is limited.

Overall, orbital radiotherapy generally causes a reduction in soft tissue inflammation and an improvement in muscle function, proposes and optic neuropathy. The effects on proptosis and ophthalmoplegia are usually not sufficient and patients may still need orbital decompression and strabismus surgery. However, radiation may shorten the interval before surgery can be performed.

Louise, who had orbital radiotherapy for her Graves' ophthalmopathy one month after developing symptoms of congestive GO, noticed significant improvement within four months after the completion of her treatments. She is quick to add, though, that she may have experienced improvement without radiotherapy since she experienced spontaneous remission from Graves' disease after using ATDs for only two months, followed by six months of complementary therapy. She had no adverse complications or side effects from the orbital radiotherapy. A decade after her orbital radiotherapy she remains free of symptoms.

Writing in *Endocrine Emergencies*, Dr. Yeatts reports that, in his experience, patients who have undergone orbital radiation therapy before orbital decompression respond less favorably when it comes to proptosis because the resulting fibrotic orbital tissue fails to expand into the space provided by the surgery. This could necessitate additional eye muscle surgery.

Side Effects

Although orbital radiation has few adverse effects, it can cause transient worsening of soft-tissue inflammation and loss of hair at the temples. In one study, 29 percent of patients who had orbital radiation required one or more surgeries to correct strabismus. However, Dr. Soparkar, a Houston ophthalmologist who specializes in the treatment of GO, cautions that this statistic may be misleading because many patients with congestive GO eventually do need strabismus surgery whether they have external beam radiation therapy or not.

Both retinopathy and cataracts have also been reported to occur after orbital radiotherapy. Radiation retinopathy is an extremely rare complication although it is more likely to occur in patients with systemic microvascular disease related to diabetes mellitus because retinopathy may occur spontaneously in patients with diabetes mellitus. Although long-term studies do not support an increased risk of tumors, orbital radiotherapy is not recommended for patients younger than 30 years old.

One long-term study by S.D. Marques and his colleagues involving 453 patients who had orbital radiotherapy concluded that orbital radiotherapy is safe and effective for the treatment of GO. The study's authors concluded that the overall response rate in these patients was 96 percent, with a 98 percent patient satisfaction rate. No irreparable long-term effects were noted. The most common late effect was cataract development, and this tended to occur more frequently in older patients and was treatable. Although improvement has been noted after one to four weeks, the full effects of orbital radiation are reported to take up to six months to show up, and for this reason, the authors recommended that surgery be postponed until the peak effects of orbital radiotherapy had been achieved.

Another recent study performed at the Mayo Clinic involving 42 patients showed no benefits from orbital radiotherapy when patients were seen at three and six-month follow-up visits. Six months after radiotherapy patients showed no evidence of clinically or statistically significant benefits. Furthermore, patients treated six months earlier in the course of their illness showed similar results. Previous steroid therapy also had no effect on outcome. Because this is an extremely small study of a limited population that has been widely criticized for its methodology, further studies confirming this would be needed before one could conclude that orbital radiotherapy is without benefits.

Orthoptics

Orthoptics is a special field of ophthalmology that specializes in disorders of vision: binocular vision (use of both eyes together), eye movements and nystagmus (uncontrolled eye movements). Patients with diplopia and related disorders often consult orthoptists (practitioners of orthoptics) to manage their conditions. Orthoptists often work in cooperation with ophthalmologists, neuro-ophthalmologists and endocrinologists.

Orthoptic examinations and treatment play an important role in the rehabilitation of patients with diplopia. Diagnostic tests used in orthoptics include: OKN; Doll's Head Maneuver; prism and cover testing; clinical and formal EOG assessment of saccadic velocities; binocular visual field testing; Hess/Lees Screen; forced ductions; forced generations; EMG; differential IOP; Tensilon; and dynamic MRI testing.

Orbital Surgery

Patients with GO may require one or more orbital surgeries. However, surgery is not used as often as it was in the past. Now that it is known that GO follows a natural course and is self-limiting, surgery is generally used as a last resort and only when the optic nerve is compromised, corneal exposure is severe or there is a significant limitation of ocular motility as a consequence of extreme proptosis.

Many insurance companies require second opinions or pre-admission authorizations for orbital surgery. Therefore, it is important to check with your insurance provider ahead of time. Also, aspirin, and other medications that interfere with blood clotting, including some Vitamin E and certain herbal preparations, should be avoided for one week before surgery. A friend who was initially told that insurance would not cover her surgery, insisting that it was merely cosmetic, reported that the insurance company changed its mind after seeing before and after pictures that clearly showed the differences in appearance caused by proptosis.

It is also important to check with your physician in the weeks before surgery for a list of pre-operative requirements, including dietary restrictions. At your pre-operative visit, your doctor will also discuss the timeframe of your recovery and the type of anesthesia he or she plans to administer.

The three most common surgeries used for GO include: 1) orbital decompression; 2) eye muscle surgery; and 3) eyelid surgery. If all three surgeries are performed, the sequence is: orbital decompression, eye muscle surgery, and then eyelid surgery.

Orbital Decompression

Orbital decompression is indicated whenever the therapeutic goal is expansion of the orbital volume; for instance, in compressive optic neuropathy. In this condition, apical decompression is the goal and it serves to relieve the crowded orbital apex (the rear portion of the orbit). For patients with significant proptosis with exposure keratitis, orbital decompression allows the globe to settle more posteriorly (further back) and often slightly more inferiorly or downward, improving the position of the lower lid and decreasing corneal exposure.

The greatest advantage of orbital decompression remains its potential to restore vision immediately to those patients whose vision is threatened or compromised. Orbital decompression is particularly helpful in patients who have symptoms that respond poorly to medical management, such as proptosis, with or without extraocular muscle imbalance, and exposure keratopathy. Corneal ulceration resulting from severe proptosis is also an indication for orbital decompression.

However, orbital decompression has advanced little in the past 100 years. Dr. Robert Goldberg, writing in the *Archives of Ophthalmology*, says that his own outlook has changed in the last decade due to current knowledge of the autoimmune nature of GO. He writes that our understanding of the natural history of GO and its management in the non-inflammatory vs. inflammatory phase has made surgery for optic neuropathy less common. Also, improved surgical techniques have allowed for more aggressive treatment for proptosis when it is warranted. Furthermore, patients today are more likely to request surgery for the cosmetic changes caused by GO after the disease has resolved.

Orbital Decompression Procedure

Decompression refers to a mechanism used to reduce compression or congestion. There are four bony surfaces of the orbit that are available for decompression:

1. The medial wall overlying the ethmoid (relating to the upper nasal cavity) sinuses. The posterior (rear) medial wall that overlies the apical portion of the muscles just anterior to the annulus of Zinn is often used when optic neuropathy is present.

2. The floor of the orbit, overlying the maxillary (near the middle section of the nose) sinus.

3. The anterior lateral wall that includes the zygoma (along the sides of the face below the orbit) surrounding the anterior tip of the inferior orbital fissure, which can be decompressed out to temporalis muscle and buccal fat. This is the classic method and typically provides approximately 2 mm of orbital volume.

4. The deep lateral wall. This consists of the bulk of the greater wing of the sphenoid, which is composed of thick bone in the area between the inferior and superior orbital fissure including the fossa of the lacrimal gland. Decompression in this area is limited due to the temporalis muscle fascia and by the dura or outer layer of the anterior and middle cranial fossa. Removal of the deep lateral wall can be performed extracranially through cosmetically hidden incisions.

A. Orbital Septurm — layer holding back orbital fat
B. Levator Aponeurosis — eyelid muscle tendon seen through septum

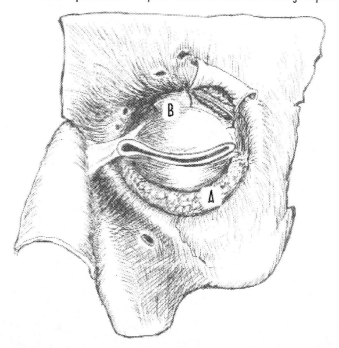

The Eyelid and Facial Muscles. Illustrated by Marvin G. Miller. Copyright © Elaine A. Moore. Reprinted with permission.

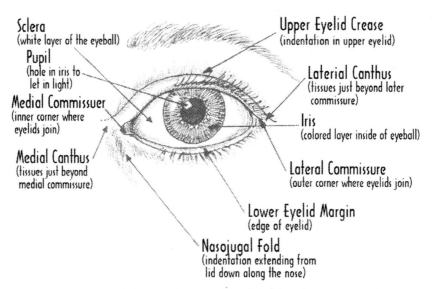

Sclera
(white layer of the eyeball)

Pupil
(hole in iris to let in light)

Medial Commissuer
(inner corner where eyelids join)

Medial Canthus
(tissues just beyond medial commissure)

Upper Eyelid Crease
(indentation in upper eyelid)

Laterial Canthus
(tissues just beyond later commissure)

Iris
(colored layer inside of eyeball)

Lateral Commissure
(outer corner where eyelids join)

Lower Eyelid Margin
(edge of eyelid)

Nasojugal Fold
(indentation extending from lid down along the nose)

The Orbital Septum. Illustrated by Marvin G. Miller. Copyright © Elaine A. Moore. Reprinted with permission.

Orbital Walls

Orbital decompression refers to mechanisms, generally surgeries, which are used to provide more orbital space. Orbital decompression involves removing bone, and allowing the orbital soft tissues to expand into space previously taken up by bone (lateral wall or roof) or sinuses (the ethmoid and maxillary sinuses). Orbital compression surgery varies depending on the number of walls removed. The more walls removed, the more resulting space (although surgery involving all four walls is rarely performed).

A two-wall decompression allows expansion of the orbit into actual rather than potention spaces, and allows for decompression of the orbital apex in patients with optic neuropathy. The superior (transfrontal) approach removes the roof of the orbit, but it is rarely used today because of the associated risks, including intracerebral hemorrhage, damage to the frontal lobe, and meningitis.

The orbital floor and medial wall can be approached transorbitally through the eyelid or transantrally through the gingival sulcus. The latter method allows greater exposure of the orbital apex, facilitating decompression in compressive optic neuropathy.

The inferior (transantral) approach, which has been modified to remove the lateral wall as well as the floor and medial wall of the orbit, is most often performed today. The advantage of this approach is that this surgery leaves no external scar, and decompression is very effective (averaging a 4.7 mm decrease in proptosis).

Removal of the floor and medial wall can also be accomplished by an anterior approach through a transconjunctival or translid incision. This procedure is reported to reduce the risk of developing postoperative diplopia although it may worsen pre-existing diplopia.

Removal of portions of three walls (floor, lateral and medial) can be accomplished by either combining transantral or translid decompression with lateral decompression or by means of the coronal approach. In the coronal approach, a skin-muscle incision is made from ear to ear behind the hair border and the lateral wall, and most of the ethmoid and medial portion of the floor are removed. This approach is reported to cause greater reduction of diplopia and a smaller risk of diplopia.

Orbital Fat Orbitotomy

A similar approach is to remove orbital fat through medial-upper and lateral-lower anterior orbitotomy. Although the reduction in proptosis is generally less, side effects are limited to temporary motility impairment of the inferior oblique muscle. In recent years, decompression has also been accomplished by removing intraconal orbital fat in cases characterized by enlargement of the fat compartment as opposed to primarily extraocular muscle enlargement.

There are a number of different techniques for incisions, some of which are associated with visible scarring. In general, hidden incisions are preferable and include the endoscopic transnasal, medial conjunctival, inferior conjunctival, eyelid crease, and transcoronal incisions.

Extended Pterional Orbit Decompression

The main indications for this procedure are: compressive optic neuropathy with progressive visual loss; exposure keratopathy; malignant, disfiguring exophthalmos; severe orbital inflammation with pain; and increasing strabismus.

In the extended procedure the skin is incised 1 cm behind the hairline starting at the preauricular region. The skin flap is turned anteriorly until the region of the zygomatic process of the frontal bone, and the frontal process of the zygoma are visible. Aided by a microscope, the surgeon removes the greater wing of the sphenoid bone; the upper bony border of the superior orbital fissure and the lateral half of the orbital roof;

and the lower and lateral borders of the superior orbital fissure. After removal of the lateral parts of the bony orbital roof, the periosteum of the orbit is incised, allowing orbital contents to expand into the newly created orbital space. At the end of the procedure, the temporal muscle is reflected back into position and sutured.

A. Lateral Canthal Tendon — tendon anchoring lids to bone
B. Lower Tarus (Tarsal Plate) — stiffening element (like cartilage)
C. Levator Muscle — main opening muscle of upper lid
D. Superior Oblique Tendon — tendon of muscle moving the eyeball
E. Inferior Oblique Muscle — muscle moving the eyeball
F. Lacrimal Gland (Tear Gland)— gland that produces watery tears
G. Lacrimal Sac (Tear Sac) — part of the tear drainage system
H. Fat — orbital fat which extends into the eyelids
I. Orbital Rim — rim of the socket bone

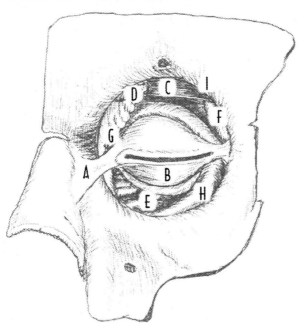

*Facial and Eyelid Anatomy. Illustrated by Marvin G. Miller. Copyright ©
Elaine A. Moore. Reprinted with permission.*

Pros and Cons of Orbital Decompression

While orbital decompression surgery offers a mechanical resolution, it does not affect the disease process itself. That is, although orbital decompression is effective in increasing orbital space, it doesn't modify the inflammatory autoimmune aspect of Graves' ophthalmopathy. In the active stages of the disease, deposits of GAG and lymphocyte cell infiltration may again compress the increased orbital space, requiring additional surgery. This is the reason decompression surgery is only performed during the active disease stage when vision is compromised.

Complications of transantral two-wall decompression include transient intraorbital anesthesia (temporary paralysis in the eye area), diplopia, nasolacrimal tear duct obstruction, and sinusitis. Diplopia is considered the major disadvantage to orbital decompression surgery because it may affect up to two-thirds of patients who didn't have diplopia before surgery.

Diplopia occurs because surgery may create a new condition of strabismus or exacerbate (worsen) existing oculomotor (eye muscle movement) dysfunction. A restrictive vertical strabismus may sometimes result from entrapment of orbital contents, including extraocular muscles, in the decompression site. Neuroimaging is helpful in confirming this if this complication is suspected. If entrapment has occurred, a qualified oculoplastic surgeon can perform orbital exploratory surgery to release adhesions before strabismus repair is performed.

Orbital Fat Decompression

As an alternative to orbital bone decompression, surgeons at Columbia-Presbyterian Medical Center in New York have successfully used orbital fat decompression to treat dysthyroid optic neuropathy in five patients (eight orbits). This procedure, which was performed by Dr. Michael Kazim and medical team, was described in the *British Journal of Ophthalmology*. In all cases, optic neuropathy was reversed, and there were no cases of postoperative diplopia, enophthalmos, globe ptosis, or anaesthesia at the one-year follow-up examination.

The study's authors report that when medical therapy—either steroids or orbital radiotherapy—is ineffective, orbital fat decompression is an effective solution for decreasing orbital pressure. In this procedure, incisions were made in both the upper and lower eyelids. The orbital septum was opened and prolapsing orbital fat was removed by using blunt surgical dissection deep into the orbit. Electrocautery was used to cut fat and coagulate blood vessels in the area. An average of 3–6 ml of fat was removed through the lower compartment, and 2 ml was removed through the superior fat compartment. The incisions were closed with nylon sutures that were removed five days after surgery. Patients were observed in the hospital for 24 hours and treated with ice packs.

Eye Muscle Surgery

Extraocular muscle surgery is used in an effort to correct misalignment of the eyes and reduce diplopia. In diploplia, the eye muscles are out of alignment, and surgery is performed in an effort to correct alignment. While it's difficult to correct all positions of gaze in diplopia, restoration of a single binocular vision in the primary (looking straight ahead) and reading positions is considered a success. Surgery should be employed when GO is active but in a resting phase; for instance, when the muscle is inflamed, but not when fibrotic changes have occurred and scar tissue has formed.

Eye muscle surgery to correct diplopia is performed on both eyes, even though one eye may be unaffected or "good." Eye muscle surgery may release a restricted muscle, but the muscle is often still unable to move normally because of its enlargement or fibrosis. Thus, even with surgery, the more affected eye will have a very limited movement and double vision will persist unless one is looking straight ahead. By limiting the movement of the "good" eye, the surgeon can properly align the muscles and maximize the area in which one can see singly.

During surgery the muscle is cut from its attachment to the eyeball and reattached further back. The inferior rectus is the muscle that most often requires corrective surgery, followed by the medial rectus, the superior rectus, and on rare occasions, the lateral rectus. The surgical aim is to recess or free the most affected restricted muscle.

In eye muscle surgery, the eyelids are gently opened and the dysfunctional muscle identified. Skin incisions are not usually required. The incision is made in the thin white tissue overlying the muscle. The muscle is then separated from the eye and reattached in its new position using dissolvable sutures. The eye muscle may be reattached using an adjustable slipknot, which allows re-positioning or fine-tuning after the patient wakes up, and sometimes after the anesthesia has worn off.

Most eye muscle surgeries can be performed on an outpatient basis and vary from 30 minutes to two hours. Postoperative pain and nausea may occur and medications are generally prescribed to alleviate these symptoms. Combination antibiotic-steroids, such as Pred-G drops, may also be prescribed—for use twice a day for five to seven days beginning the day after surgery. Ice packs, applied for 10-20 minutes hourly, may also be prescribed to help reduce post-operative swelling and discomfort.

Strabismus surgery

In strabismus surgery, an incision is made in the tissue covering the eye, and muscles are repositioned depending on which direction the eye is turning. Recovery time is rapid, with most patients being able to resume activities within a few days. More than one surgery may be required until the problem is fully corrected.

Eyelid Surgery

Graves' ophthalmopathy often causes the eyelids to open more widely. This causes the lids to retract, which can result in excessive tearing and discomfort. Eyelid retraction is generally related to an exaggerated reaction of the superior rectus or levator muscles that might be secondary to the contracture of the inferior rectus muscle. Recession of the eyelid retractors via surgery allows the eyelid to return to its normal position. Surgery can also be used to reposition and lengthen eyelids and to remove herniated orbital fat.

Eyelid surgery (tarsorraphy) can be performed on an emergency basis in patients with exposure keratitis or corneal ulceration, but it's usually carried out for rehabilitative or cosmetic purposes to correct eyelid malposition after medical treatment or orbital decompression. Unless an emergency situation exists, surgery should be postponed until GO has been stable and inactive for four to six months. If orbital decompression, eye muscle and eyelid surgery are required, eyelid surgery is generally performed last.

Surgical upper eyelid retraction techniques include: recession of Muller's muscle; levator aponeurosis recession; levator myotomy; and temporary or permanent canthorrhaphy. For lower lid retraction, the most effective technique involves recession of the lid retractors followed by the insertion of a scleral spacer. Spacer elements of hard palate, auricular cartilage, or preserved cadaveric sclera may all be inserted to help in repositioning the eyelid.

Blepharoplasty

Patients with droopy eyelids or eyebrows often develop headaches because they're forced to involuntarily raise their eyebrows and use their forehead muscles to allow additional light to enter their eyes. Blepharoplasty is a surgical procedure used to remove unnecessary fat and skin in this area. This technique is often used to remove under-eye "bags."

Insurance Concerns

Upper eyelid surgery is usually covered by medical insurance. However, it's important that the patient undergoes specific tests, such as peripheral vision testing, before surgery is performed to establish a baseline level. Tests performed after surgery will show a difference, demonstrating that surgery was needed. As I previously mentioned, my friend Mary, a college professor in Minnesota, was initially denied pre-authorization for eyelid surgery. Along with her request to have her case re-evaluated, she sent her insurance company pictures of herself before and after developing Graves' disease. This was enough to convince her insurance company that surgery was warranted and they honored her claim.

Experimental and New Therapies

Anti-Cytokine Treatment

Cytokines are potent immune system chemicals released during the immune response. Cytokines are known to modulate the immune response, and they perpetuate the disease process in GO. Biological agents aimed at blocking the effects of cytokines, particularly TNF-α and IL-1, are currently being studied for their use in treating GO. Those biological agents under investigation include cytokine receptor antagonists, monoclonal antibodies to cytokines, soluble cytokine receptors and counter-regulatory cytokines.

In clinical studies conducted in vitro, that is, in test tubes, GAG synthesis and GO progression appear to be inhibited by the administration of the soluble IL-1 receptor and IL-1 receptor antagonist. However, patient data is lacking.

Botox

Many people are familiar with Botox (botulinum toxin A) because of its ability to firm wrinkled tissue, but few people know that Botox has medical applications. Botox (40 U given as an injection) has been successfully used as an alternative to strabismus eye muscle surgery and in eyelid surgery. To correct strabismus, the drug is injected into the eye muscle to temporarily paralyze the muscle. This allows the opposite muscle to tighten and straighten the eye. While the effects of Botox wear off after several weeks, on some occasions this allows adequate time for muscle alignment.

In eyelid surgery, Botox may be injected into the glabelar muscles, corrugator supercilii, and sometimes the procerus, to induce a flattening of the glabelar region and improvement of the medial eyebrow contour and glabelar furrowing. The use of Botox alone may also be considered an alternative to eyelid surgery in the rehabilitation of patients with upper lid retraction and overacting protractors resulting in a thyroid frown.

Bromocriptine

The drug bromocriptine has also been studied for its benefits in GO, which are reported to be similar to other conventional therapies. The effects of bromocriptine are related to its possible anti-proliferative effect on potentially autoreactive T lymphocytes. Bromocriptine (Parlodel) is an ergot derivative with potent dopamine receptor agonist activity, which is commonly used to inhibit prolactin secretion.

Metronidazole

The anti-parasitic drug metronidazole has also been studied for its effects on GO. A transient benefit was noted in one study, but more studies are needed before the efficacy of this agent can be established.

11
COMPLEMENTARY THERAPY IN GO

Similar to most disorders of an autoimmune nature, GO shows a favorable response to dietary changes, stress reduction techniques, mild exercise, immunomodulators, dietary supplements (particularly antioxidant vitamins), herbal medicine and an avoidance of environmental triggers such as cigarette smoke. In severe GO, these changes are unlikely to eliminate the need for aggressive conventional treatments. But incorporating these holistic suggestions may help facilitate the response to conventional treatment.

Taking Charge

It's important for patients with GO to take an active role in their own healing process. Patients need to know that their lifestyle and dietary habits can play an important role and have an important bearing on their success in healing. Patients with symptoms of dry eye need to avoid fans and gusty winds, and they need to protect their eyes from the elements. Just as importantly, patients need to know the important role of fresh fruits, particularly berries, in achieving eye health. Patients also need to know that refined sugars and saturated fat cause immune system changes that promote inflammation. Degenerative changes in the eye often begin by middle age, and many of these changes can be prevented with lifestyle modification.

Self-Care

The following suggestions are helpful for reducing symptoms associated with GO:

- Use a blindfold over ointment-filled eyes at night. Blindfolds similar to the ones provided by airlines that flip up are particularly useful.
- Tilt the head of the bed up several inches at night.
- Use additional pillows (unless they aggravate neck problems.)
- Wear treated or tinted lenses to help reduce computer glare.
- Use a humidifier.
- Avoid allergens, using an air cleaner if dust and pets cause problems.
- Apply cool, sliced cucumbers to closed eyes.
- Apply cool tea bags seeped in German tea to closed eyes.
- Take antioxidant vitamins.
- Avoid fluorescent lights if they bother your eyes.
- Avoid fans and drafts.
- Drink at least eight glasses of water daily.
- Avoid sugars and saturated fats since they promote inflammation.
- Blink often to bathe your eyes.
- Exercise your eyes daily to prevent muscle stiffness, moving the eyes up and down, from side to side, and from near to distant objects.
- Add light exercise or meditation to your daily routine.

Antioxidants

Orally ingested antioxidants and anti-glycating agents, such as carnosine, help to prevent and treat eye disease. Although diminished blood flow to the eyes can sometimes inhibit the effects of orally ingested supplements, increasing blood antioxidant levels has been reported to show favorable effects. The antioxidants that showed the most benefits include carotene, lycopene and lutein. These antioxidants are found in orange and yellow vegetables, egg yolks, and tomatoes. Other antioxidants that showed improvement in eye health include Vitamins C and E, zinc.

A small pilot study in Greece that involved 11 patients with GO, all smokers, demonstrated an 82 percent improvement rate in patients treated with oral administration of the anti-gout medication allopurinol (300 mg daily) and the B vitamin nicotinamide (300 mg daily). A reduction of soft tissue inflammation was the most prominent finding, and no side effects of treatment were observed.

Dietary Changes

For successful healing in GO, certain dietary changes are essential. Because saturated fats and refined sugar cause immune system changes that promote inflammation, they should be avoided. Other substances to avoid included refined food, dairy products, alcohol, fatty meats, tobacco, recreational drugs and processed foods.

It is always a good idea to eat a diet rich in whole grains, green, leafy vegetables and roots, fresh fruits (especially berries and pineapple), sea vegetables, nuts and seeds, beans, shiitake and reishi mushroom, and low-fat white fish. A nutrient-rich diet with adequate, but not excess, protein is essential for immune system health. Because patients with thyroid disease are likely to have deficiencies of essential fatty acids, it is also important to add omega oil supplements. Flaxseed oil, taken in 500 mg capsules twice daily, is reported to benefit patients with congestive GO.

Herbal Medicine

Herbs used to lower thyroid hormone levels, such as *Lycopus virginicus* (bugleweed), *Leonurus cardiaca* (motherwort) and *Melissa officianalis* (lemon balm), can reduce symptoms of GO by bringing thyroid hormone levels into the normal range. Bugleweed is also reported to inhibit the immune system's production of thyroid antibodies, thereby helping reduce symptoms of congestive GO.

Extracts of milk thistle, both *Silybum marianum* and *Silibinin*, are used in traditional Chinese medicine to reduce symptoms in GO. Herbalists will prescribe herbs in the form of tonics with ingredients based on one's individual constitution and symptoms. In Japanese herbal medicine, the tonic minor bupleurum decoction is used as a complementary agent for patients with GO who are using prednisone.

At the First Affiliated Hospital of Guanzhou Traditional Chinese Medicine University, researchers have successfully used the herb Jiayanxiao (JYX) in conjunction with methimazole to treat exophthalmos in patients with GO. In one published study, the total improvement rate in the treated group was 80.6 percent compared to a control group with an improvement rate of 50 percent.

Other herbs reported to be beneficial for treating immune disorders include garlic, cumin, turmeric, green tea, cinnamon, mint and chamomile.

Always consult with a naturopathic physician or an herbalist before beginning a complementary program involving herbal therapies.

Jolethin

Jolethin, a compound containing iodine and lecithin, produced by the Dai-Ichi pharmaceutical manufacturing company in Japan, is used for the treatment of Graves' hyperthyroidism and Graves' ophthalmopathy. The daily dose is equivalent to 100 mcg of iodine and the compound is less subject to deterioration than other forms of iodine.

Psychoneuroimmunology

In the 1950's, when Hans Selye proved that the stress response damages health, our ideas about a healthy lifestyle began to change. When Dr. Norman Cousins cured his own autoimmune disease, ankylosing spondylitis (a particularly destructive type of arthritis), with humor and biofeedback, the scientific world began to put the pieces together.

In the 1980's, Harvard researchers proved that the immune system, the nervous system and the endocrine system all influenced one another. The stress of bereavement, for example, may cause more overt nervous system symptoms, but both the endocrine glands and the immune system cells are profoundly affected. The scientific discipline that studies the inner-workings of these three systems is known as psychoneuroimmunology or PNI.

Stress Reduction

Besides causing heart problems and stomach ailments, stress damages the immune system. Although the initial effects may not be obvious, stress plays a major role in both triggering autoimmune diseases and causing symptoms to flare up. Studies show that stress reduction techniques, such as yoga, tai chi, biofeedback, and meditation, cause immune system changes that reduce inflammation and inhibit the activity of autoreactive cells. Dr. Charles Soparkar, a Houston ophthalmologist, has observed that stress significantly contributes to a worsening of symptoms in GO. Stress is also reported to be the most common trigger for Graves' disease and is known to cause immune system changes that promote autoantibody production.

Immune System Balance

People with autoimmune disorders are thought to have immune systems that are weak as a result of stress, poor diets, recent infections or compromised health. The normal balance between suppressor and helper cells becomes disrupted. This causes the immune system to work ineffectively. And, consequently, immune system cells over-react to foreign antigens and produce auto-reactive lymphocytes. These cells trigger changes in other cells, inducing a process that leads to the development of autoantibodies. The autoantibodies, in term, cause disease symptoms such as inflammation.

Avoiding sugars, saturated fats and allergens promotes immune system health. Patients who are unable to limit their exposure to allergens should use prescription medicines that amend the immune response. And while light exercise is essential for immune system health, extended periods of strenuous exercise can be detrimental to our immune systems.

While stress is a normal part of life and essential for creativity, our reaction to stress or our exposure to chronic stress can weaken and damage our immune systems. Exercises and techniques that reduce stress and help us to adapt to stressful situations are important in any natural program designed to limit symptoms of GO.

Immunomodulators

Our goal is to have a strong healthy immune system. To achieve this, we need to avoid immune system stimulants, like the herbs Echinacea and Ashwaganda, because these stimulants encourage immune system cells to over-react to both foreign and self antigens, and we need to avoid or control immune system stressors such as sugar, aspartame, caffeine, alcohol and stress itself. Immune systems that are hyperactive or underactive are weak and ineffective. A hyperactive immune system elicits changes that contribute to autoimmunity, allergies, and inflammation. Sustained periods of hyperimmunity may lead to immune exhaustion and collapse.

Immunomodulators are natural substances that work to balance the immune system. They're able to strengthen weak and sluggish immune systems and slow down immune systems that are overactive. In studies, immunomodulators have also been shown to counteract the natural immune system depression caused by strenuous exercise.

The best-known immunomodulators include plant sterols and sterolins. These compounds are chemicals derived from plant fats such as beta sitosterol. While sterols are present in waxy vegetables, cooking destroys them. And when vegetables are frozen, the sterols and sterolins are destroyed during the process of thawing.

Plant sterols and sterolins are found in the commercial product Sterinol, which can be found in most health food stores. Sterinol is sold in 20 mg capsules that can be used up to three times daily. Sterols are also found in the Polynesian plant *Morinda citrifolia* (Noni, Nonu, Nono). Sterols should not be used in patients who have had tissue or organ transplants.

Other immunomodulators include:

- Reishi mushroom extract (*Gonderma lucidum, Ganoderma*) sold as the plant extract or in products listed as glycocentials.
- German chamomile (*Matricaria recutita*) used as a tea (up to 3 gm daily or 6–8 capsules containing 500 mg of herbal extract).
- Flower pollen extract (Cernitin and Prostaphil patent preparations), used in servings of 240 mg of the water soluble extract or 12 mg of the oil soluble extract, which are found in capsule or tablet forms.
- Glyconutrients, described in the following section.

Dietary Supplements

Healing Sugars

Healing sugars are natural saccharides that were once plentiful in our food supply. These sugars are essential for health in that they strengthen and balance the immune system.

Because of changes in food technology and processing, many people are deficient in these sugars, which are known as glyconutrients. The eight healing sugars include: mannose; glucose; galactose; xylose; fucose; N-acetylglucosamine; N-acetylgalactosamine; and N-acetylneuraminic acid. Only two of these sugars, glucose (found in plants and table sugar) and galactose (found in milk and certain fruit pectins), are common in today's diet. Note: fructose (found in fruits and table sugar) is not an essential sugar.

Glyconutrients help the body heal. Glucosamine, a natural metabolic product of the essential saccharide N-acetylglucosamine, is widely prescribed today for arthritis. In autoimmune diseases, helper T cells are generally increased, whereas suppressor T cells are low in number. Glyconutrients help restore the proper balance in these cells, thereby helping the immune system function effectively. Glyconutrients also help in reducing inflammation.

In human and animal studies, glyconutrients have been shown to improve the balance of the various lymphocytes and reduce autoimmune symptoms. Some researchers believe that defects in sugar metabolism caused by a lack of essential glyconutrients contribute to autoimmune disease development.

Interested in this report, I began using glyconutrient supplements nine months ago. I began using one teaspoon of Ambrotose by Mannatech and after three months began taking two teaspoons. Although I did not notice immediate improvement, after three weeks I noticed a reduction of inflammation. Blood tests also showed a decrease in my titers of thyroid antibodies and more stable thyroid function tests.

Bee Pollen

Bee pollen, taken in the form of granules, has also been reported to reduce symptoms in GO. Most of the healing properties of herbs have been studied informally and can be found in the lore of folk medicine. Dr. H.C.A. Vogel, writing in *The Nature Doctor* originally published in 1950 in Switzerland, describes the benefits of bee pollen for GO. He cautions that patients with Graves' disease should wait until their symptoms of thyrotoxicosis are under control before using bee pollen because it may raise blood pressure. Unfortunately, although there's a great deal of anecdotal evidence, there are no reported double-blind studies to support these facts.

Riboflavin, Vitamin B2

John Johnson, a physicist and founder of the website *www.ithyroid.com* recommends using Riboflavin (Vitamin B2) to relieve symptoms of dry eye, particularly foreign body sensation. Although as a general rule, the B vitamins should be balanced, Johnson found improvement after increasing his B2 intake. Even though he was already taking supplements equivalent to more than ten times the minimum daily requirement, he was experiencing eye symptoms similar to those associated with Riboflavin deficiency. Johnson also reports that an excess amount of other B vitamins, especially thiamine (Vitamin B1) upsets the balance and contributes to riboflavin deficiency. Besides increasing his daily intake of B2, he reduced his intake of the other B vitamins before he experienced optimal results.

Energy Healing

Energy healing is a welcome addition to any complementary therapies plan. Some forms of this discipline include acupuncture, acupressure, moxibustion and bright light therapy. Energy healing has a long history and developed in many diverse cultures at different times. The basis of energy healing is that people have a vital life force known as *ch'i* or *qi*. From this source, energy travels to other parts of the body. Disruptions or blockages of the body's energy flow lead to imbalance, characterized by an accumulation of toxins and poor health. Energy healing is used to both diagnose and correct these imbalances.

Eye Exercises

My friend Jody's ophthalmologist recommended these exercises for her. They're intended to correct diplopia and tone eye muscles. Jody's experiences with GO are included in the next chapter.

1. Find a focal point on the wall or somewhere in front of you. Look up HARD and hold for five seconds—do a set of five of these. Repeat, looking to the left, then to the right and finally look downward. Always hold for five seconds and do five sets. In the beginning these exercises may make your eyes ache, but that's a GOOD thing—it means you're stretching the eye muscles. This is essential for limbering them up and getting them working together again. Repeat this exercise two to three times daily.

2. Roll your eyes SLOWLY, all the way around, trying hard to make both eyes work together. This may not be easy in the beginning, but it gets easier as the muscles limber up. I roll them in one direction, rest for a few seconds then roll them in the other direction. Repeat this exercise two to three times daily.

3. This one is one I work on, but haven't yet accomplished. I use a pen (for me it is easier to use a white pen with a red cap). Hold the pen out in front of you at arms' length, then slowly bring it back towards the nose, trying to cross the eyes. As soon as you feel the eyes split or separate, start over. Do this in sets of five, several times a day.

These exercises sound like they might take a lot of time, but they really don't take long once you make them a habit. The reason we develop double vision is because our eyes no longer work in tandem. One of the eyes may have a muscle that's "shortened up" because of the eye disease; these exercises can help to lengthen and tone the affected muscle, improving diplopia. For example, Jody noticed a lessening of her diplopia after just eight days.

12

PSYCHOSOCIAL FACTORS: THE SURVIVORS

The psychological and social effects of GO have long been recognized. One friend, Jenny, a health professional in her mid-thirties, stated that GO robbed her of her best years. For the past ten years she's suffered from the effects of GO, and she's endured five different corrective surgical procedures. Although she recently became engaged, she bitterly regrets the bleak years during which she had "no social life."

The effects of GO can distort facial expressions, causing patients to feel self-conscious. When patients with GO develop hostile or startled expressions, their social interactions may suffer. Jane, an elementary school teacher in her late forties, reported that her proptosis affected her relationships with her students. Afraid of upsetting them, she avoided close interaction. Before she had corrective surgery, Jane used to wake up early each morning to see how her eyes looked. When her eyes looked particularly bad, she stayed home.

In recent years several different research groups have formally studied the psychosocial effects of living with GO. The following section discusses the results of these studies.

Study Results

To evaluate psychosocial changes related to GO, researchers at the University of Amsterdam in the Netherlands developed a quality-of-life questionnaire that measures health-related quality-of-life issues. Study subjects were tested before and after having corrective treatment for GO. Overall, subjects reported higher quality-of-life scores after treatment, particularly after corrective rehabilitative surgery.

Researchers in Mainz, Germany devised a similar study, designed to assess the impact of GO on quality-of-life. Using a questionnaire referred to as the "Medical Outcomes Study (MOS)," researchers questioned patients with varying degrees of GO severity. Compared to a large reference or normal control group, patients with GO had low scores, indicating an impaired quality-of-life. Significant differences from the control group were seen in vitality, social functioning, mental health, health perceptions and bodily pain. Significantly, the degree of difference wasn't related to disease severity but to the fact that they had noticeable cosmetic changes.

A similar study conducted at the Combined Thyroid Eye Clinic Newcastle Hospitals in England also documented alterations in the psychological and social functioning of patients with GO. Patients were questioned about personality traits, anxiety and depression, general health, coping strategies, mood alterations and self-consciousness. Results of this study showed a direct correlation between disease severity and depression. Patients with more severe GO also reported that they'd become more introverted, particularly in social settings.

Of all the symptoms reported, exophthalmos had the greatest impact on reported mood alterations. Incidental findings included the fact that patients with GO were reportedly more likely to be cigarette smokers. However, cigarette consumption fell dramatically after the patients were diagnosed with GO. Patients with GO also reported lower alcohol intake after their diagnosis, which was related to their reduced social interaction.

Stories of Survivors

The follow testimonies are true accounts of patients with GO. These patients have volunteered to share their stories to help readers understand the effects of GO on a personal level. In some instances, the names or demographics of the patient have been changed to protect their identities. Each of these patients is a genuine survivor. All of these patients have taken the time to learn the intricacies of their condition; they've forged good working relationships with their doctors; and they've worked closely with their physicians to choose therapies best suited for them.

Jody

My friend Jody was diagnosed with Graves' disease in May 1996 after being hospitalized for hypertension, arrhythmia and congestive heart failure as well as other symptoms suggestive of thyroid storm. While she was in the hospital, her doctor did not run thyroid tests. He merely gave her medications to control her cardiac symptoms. Home from the hospital, she suspected she might be hyperthyroid and consulted a different doctor. He ran the appropriate tests and found that she did indeed have severe Graves' disease. This doctor referred Jody to an endocrinologist.

Jody's Treatment Options

The specialist with whom she consulted insisted that Jody was too sick to be treated with anti-thyroid drugs. She warned Jody and her family that she needed to have aggressive treatment as soon as possible. While Jody and her husband discussed their options, her doctor warned her that surgery was too risky, leaving RAI ablation as the only option.

Jody recalls the doctor saying "You'll swallow a little bit of radioactive material in capsule form. Afterwards, you'll take one little pill a day for the rest of your life. In six months, you'll feel so good you'll realize just how sick you've been." She also told Jody that she was lucky to have no signs of eye disease, and that by being treated with RAI, she would never have to deal with GO. Jody had RAI one month later after being prescribed PTU and propranolol (Inderal) for only 30 days despite the fact that it takes six to eight weeks for PTU to show its maximum effects.

The Aftermath

Soon after her ablation, Jody realized that her doctor hadn't been entirely honest. Seven years after RAI, Jody has fired two endocrinologist and two primary doctors who kept her hypothyroid, and she's also fired one eye doctor. Jody describes the first four years after RAI as "hypohell." She suffered from joint pain, muscle aches, hair loss, depression and tremendous weight gain. Her doctors monitored her with a TSH test alone and insisted that her symptoms were not thyroid-related. They suggested she take Prozac for the anxiety and depression (which are common symptoms of hypothyroidism). The doctors never mentioned that thyroid function might be the cause of these symptoms. But, Jody writes, all of these symptoms were virtually nothing compared to her experiences with GO.

After joining an online support group, Jody learned that she should also be monitored for thyroid hormone levels. When she insisted that her doctor run a FT4 and FT3 level, the first primary doctor refused so she added them to the lab requisition on her own. Her doctor was surprised at how low her levels were. He increased the 0.075 mcg of levothyroxine that she'd been on for four years to 0.088 mcg.

When Jody eventually consulted a new doctor, her dose was immediately raised to 0.112 mcg and, later, 0.125 mcg, but her T3 was still low due to a conversion problem. (Note: Current research shows that in some laboratory methods for TSH, there are interferences from TSH receptor antibodies, which cause falsely decreased TSH results.)

Without measurements of her thyroid hormone levels, Jody would have never received proper treatment for her thyroid condition. The new doctor that Jody consulted and continues to see applauds Jody's efforts to learn all that she can. And this doctor always welcomes the abstracts and articles that Jody brings her.

Jody's Poor Eyes

Two years later, in the spring of 2000, Jody realized that her eyes—which had become puffy and dry after RAI—were getting worse. Her first doctor blamed it on allergies. Her endocrinologist referred her to an ophthalmologist. At the time of her first appointment in July of 2000, Jody had very active GO, with symptoms of diplopia, blurred vision, lid lag, loss of night vision, increased intraocular pressure, severe light sensitivity accompanied by pain, loss of peripheral vision, and mild proptosis. Jody's ophthalmologist immediately ordered a TSI level. Her level was 199 percent (normal is less than 130 percent), indicating that she was still producing the antibodies that cause hyperthyroidism in Graves' disease. Only now they were attacking her orbital tissues. Initially, her doctors monitored her condition and waited for the symptoms to spontaneously resolve.

Jody's Plan

Jody continued to research autoimmune disorders, and decided that if she needed therapy she wanted to use anti-thyroid drugs in conjunction with thyroid replacement hormone to reduce her TSI levels. This time she knew all about treatment options, including how they worked and their side effects. She wanted to eliminate the disease right at its cause. And she knew that people using anti-thyroid drugs as a treatment for hyperthyroidism often experienced improvement in their GO.

Although her endocrinologist agreed to this plan, her ophthalmologist wanted her to use steroids or orbital radiotherapy. Jody countered. She said that if he agreed to her plan of therapy and it didn't work, she would later try a course of low dose steroids. In October 2001, Jody had a CBC (complete blood count) and liver function tests to ensure that she had no problems that would prohibit using PTU. The following report of Jody's case history written by her ophthalmologist is from September 13th, 2001.

Visual acuity: without correction 20/25 Rt. Eye, 20/40 Lt eye. On external examination she was noted to have a retraction of all four lids. Extraocular motilities demonstrated a decrease in all gazes with an oxophoria, as well as a left hypertropia. Pupils are equal, round and reactive to light and there were no afferent papillary defects noted. Conjunctiva and sclera had minimal injection.

On ocular sensory examination her Worth four dot was normal both in distance and at near, but she only demonstrated 400 seconds of steropsis. On color vision examination she answered correctly 17 out of 17 colored charts on each side. Confrontational visual fields were full on each side. Cranial nerve examination was normal except for a decrease of her extraocular motilities and a slight variation in sensation to light touch on the face. A Hertel exophthalmometry reading at a base of 93 demonstrated the right globe to be 24 mm and the left globe to be 25 mm.

On slit lamp examination the corneas were clear. Anterior chambers were deep and quiet. Irises were within normal limits. Applanation tonometry demonstrated an intraocular pressure of 23 mm of HG on the right side and 24 mm of HG on the left side. On fundus examination the discs were sharp and pink with a cup to disc ratio of 0.8. Her macula and retinal vessels were within normal limits for her age group.

Waiting for Remission

A follow-up report on October 19th, 2001 showed that spontaneous remission was currently unlikely. The report as transcribed in Jody's medical chart reads:

This is a follow-up on Jody, who, as you know, we have been following for her thyroid related orbitopathy, an exophoria, as well as a left hypertropia, her exposure keratitis, a slight ptosis and glaucoma. Acetylcholine receptor antibodies were performed and were within normal limits. Her TSI was increased to 199%. On reevaluation of 10/16/01 patient states that she experienced some slight increase of her ocular symptoms. She is having a more difficult time for close work and reading. Visual acuity without correction was 20/25 Rt eye and 20/50 Lt eye. External examination showed ptosis of the upper lids and retraction of the lower lids. Extraocular motilities were decreased. Pupils were equal, round and reactive to light, but there were no afferent papillary defects noted.

A Hertel exophthalmometry reading base of 93 demonstrated the right globe to be 24 mm and the left globe to be 25 mm. On slit lamp examination there were a few superficial punctate keratopathies present. Anterior chambers were deep and quiet. Irises were within normal limits. Applanation tonometry demonstrated an intraocular pressure of 21 mm of HG on the right side and 22 mm of HG on the left side. On fundus examination the discs were sharp and pink. At present it is our impression that Jody has the following oculoplastic diagnosis of: 1) a thyroid related orbitopathy; 2) an exophoria and a left hypertropia; 3) an exposure keratitis; 4) a slight ptosis with a negative acetylcholine receptor antibody; 5) a glaucoma suspect due to the increase of her cup to disc ratio and a slight increase of her intraocular pressure, which will continue to be followed conservatively.

In this report, the doctor also notes that Jody was advised of treatment options, including steroids and orbital radiotherapy. He notes that at present she wishes to follow a conservative course and should be reevaluated in seven to eight weeks, or sooner if the need arises. (The acetylcholine receptor antibody test is used to help diagnose myasthenia gravis, an autoimmune disorder that can cause proptosis. The negative results help in ruling out this condition.)

During this particular follow-up visit to her ophthalmologist, Jody proposed her plan of using an anti-thyroid drug (ATD) to lower her antibody levels. She knew that this would help resolve her active eye disease. Her ophthalmologist agreed but with two conditions: 1) that she use the drug propylthiouracil (PTU) because he felt that it offered better amelioration for thyroid eye disease; and 2) that her endocrinologist prescribe the appropriate dose of PTU and monitor her thyroid function while she was on it. (Her endocrinologist had already agreed to do this if the ophthalmologist was willing.) Jody was off and running to her endocrinologist, eager to begin using a non-traditional approach to healing her eye disease.

Following Her Plan

Jody began using PTU on October 28th, 2001. By November 8th, her pain had receded. By Thanksgiving Day, her diplopia was gone and she was able to drive during the daytime—something she'd been forced to give up in June of 2001. Labs drawn on Nov 11th, 2001 showed that her TSI level had dropped from 199 percent to 144 percent. Her TPO antibody levels were also still elevated. Although Jody was close to the normal range, she realized that patients who are truly not producing TSI should have levels of less than 2 percent. She made this her goal.

First Setback

However, Jody eventually became hypothyroid and had to have her thyroid hormone replacement dose increased. And in February 2002, her TSI level had risen to 177 percent. She increased her PTU to 150 mg daily taken in three divided doses. By April, her TSI levels had dropped to 110 percent, but she was still slightly hypothyroid.

A letter written by Jody's ophthalmologist dated March 27th, 2002 reports:

This is a follow-up for Jody who we are following for Graves' ophthalmopathy. The following are the results of tests from her evaluation on 3/1/02. Visual acuity: 20/25 Rt eye and 20/40 Lt eye. On external examination she was noted to have some pstosis and an improvement of the blepharitis. She was noted to have a retraction of the lower lids. Pupils were equal, round and reactive to light and there were no afferent papillary defects noted. Extraocular motilities were again decreased and she was noted to have an exophoria, as well as a left hyperphoria. Hertel exophthalmometry reading at a base of 93 demonstrated the right globe to be 25 mm and the left globe to be 26 mm. On slit lamp examination the corneas were clear. Anterior chambers were deep and quiet. Irises were within normal limits. Applanation tonometry demonstrated an intraocular pressure of 22 mm of HG on the right side and 21 mm of HG on the left side.

Thyroid Eye Disease

> On fundus examination the discs were sharp and pink with a cup to disc ratio of 0.8. Her macula and retinal vessels were within normal limits for her age group. At present it is our impression that Jody has the following oculoplastic diagnosis of: 1) a thyroid related orbitopathy; 2) an exophoria and left hyperphoria; 3) an exposure keratitis; 4) a slight ptosis with a negative acetylcholine receptor antibodies; 5) glaucoma suspect due to an increase of her intraocular pressure. To date this will continue to be followed conservatively. As you know, Jody has bee placed on PTU in an attempt to control her thyroid related orbitopathy. To date this has been slightly improved

Adjusting Her Dose

On July 7th, 2002 Jody began using a compounded T3 and T4 replacement hormone instead of a glandular extract. She'd read that the extracts could stimulate the immune system. However, the new lower dose prescription containing T3 compounded with T4 caused her to become extremely hypothyroid, and her eyes became much worse. Her right eye began to protrude more than the left, and she had a prominent stare, which she calls "the deer in the headlights look." She knew that she generally did better when she adjusted slowly to new meds, so she wanted to wait patiently before increasing her new compounded formula. However, she found herself hypothyroid at the present dose, and this was obviously a concern.

She began to call pharmacies. Although she lives in western New York State, Jody found someone at the Wellness Pharmacy—a large compounding pharmacy in Alabama—who could help her. The pharmacist she spoke to explained that T4 should never be compounded because of its half-life. By combining the two hormones into one pill, they had become attached to the matrix (meaning the filler that binds ingredients in pills together), making them both time-released. He wasn't surprised that she had become hypothyroid.

Jody then called her endocrinologist, who immediately switched her to 0.1 mg levothyroxine, and 7.5 mcg of T3 SR (taken three times daily).

Since that first week in August 2002, Jody has experienced a 100 percent turnaround. Her proptosis has receded; the diplopia (which had returned in July), is gone; and she no longer has light sensitivity. Jody is still currently tweaking her dose a bit, and is now doing well on 75 mg PTU, 0.1 mg levothyroxine and 8 mcg of T3 SR (used three times daily).

And a follow-up visit with her opthalmologist at the end of August 2002 showed remarkable improvement.

Laura

Laura, a woman from Virginia in her mid-thirties, was diagnosed with Hashimoto's thyroiditis (HT) in the summer of 1999. She'd been sick at the time, and attributed her illness to the stress of having different visitors all summer long. At the time of her diagnosis, her TSH level was 200 mu/L, with a normal or reference range of 0.4-4.5. Her total T4 level was 1.0 mcg/dl with a reference range of 5.0-14.0. Because she didn't have insurance at the time, she chose an endocrinologist she could afford. "Unfortunately," she comments, "I got my money's worth."

Four months after her diagnosis, Laura's doctor said that her Hashimoto's thyroiditis had changed. Laura was informed that she now had Hashitoxicosis. She was given this diagnosis because she'd developed symptoms of hyperthyroidism, and she now had elevated thyroid hormone levels. Her labs continued to show that she was hyperthyroid even after her dose of levothyroxine was reduced and later totally withdrawn.

This gradual move into overt hyperthyroidism suggests that she'd also moved into Graves' disease. Nearly all patients with Graves' disease have an initial period of hypothyroidism, although it may be subtle. Laura's options were outlined. Her doctor recommended RAI ablation to treat the condition he continued to call Hashitoxicosis. She opted instead for a trial of methimazole, along with a beta adrenergic blocking agent.

Laura's Eye Disease

After six continuous months of labs indicating that she was hyperthyroid, Laura began to develop signs of thyroid eye disease. She developed a prominent stare, photophobia, proptosis, and tearing. Whenever she expressed concern, her doctor would ask "Can you close your eyes?" Her answer was always yes, and this ended the discussion.

By June 2001 (about a year after the eye symptoms began), one of Laura's eyes began to swell beneath the lower lid and her proptosis worsened. Laura thought her symptoms were related to excess thyroid hormone. She wasn't told that the congestive form of GO ran its own course. A few months later, when she became eligible for medical insurance, she asked her doctor about RAI, thinking that it would fix her eye problem.

When she asked if the procedure would improve her eyes, he replied "Maybe, maybe not." He never mentioned the fact that current studies showed that it could very well worsen her eye condition. Laura asked if she needed a scan to help determine the dose of I131 she would need. He said no. It was also five weeks since her last blood tests. At that time her doctor had reduced her dose of methimazole from 20 mg to 10 mg daily.

Radioiodine Ablation

Laura's doctor gave her a list of the precautions she'd need to take for the week following RAI, but he didn't tell her whether or not she needed to continue taking her meds. He scheduled a follow-up appointment for two months after her RAI ablation. She was never cautioned to watch for symptoms of thyroid dysfunction; nor warned of her risks for both thyroid storm (a potentially fatal syndrome in which the effects of excess thyroid hormone are exaggerated) and severe hypothyroidism.

Laura was administered I131 in September of 2001. Two weeks later, her eye disease escalated to the point where she was unable to close one eye. She also developed double vision. Both eyes were swollen and she had excessive tearing. Laura's husband called her primary physician to make an appointment, and asked for a referral to an ophthalmologist. This doctor checked her thyroid hormone levels and discovered that she was already hypothyroid. She later learned that the blood work she'd had six weeks before having RAI was all well within the normal range although her dose of PTU had been reduced.

Laura's Prognosis

Because of her double vision, Laura was referred to a neuro-ophthalmologist. Before her appointment, she began researching her condition on the Internet. She emailed a neuro-ophthalmologist who'd listed his email address. His response to her query was simply this: "It is well known that RAI can worsen thyroid eye disease." She became sick when she read that, and she has been sick since—realizing that she had had a procedure she did not need, one that most likely caused her eye disease to worsen.

Laura is also upset because she had consulted a Graves' disease Internet support group early on and was told by several of the members and board moderators that RAI was very safe. No one mentioned that it could worsen her GO (although she later found out that several members of this group had had similar experiences).

Laura is currently under the care of a new endocrinologist, after firing the first doctor as well as a second. She is also being treated by a neuro-ophthalmologist and an ocular plastic surgeon. These three doctors are working together to decide what treatment course will serve her best. She continues to be on thyroid replacement hormone for her hypothyroidism, and she's learned to interpret her own laboratory results. She knows that hypothyroidism can make her condition worse.

The Waiting Game

Laura is currently waiting for her active disease phase to subside so that she can have orbital decompression surgery. The plastic surgeon, assisted by an ear, nose and throat specialist, plans to enter through her nose and remove bones between each socket and her sinus cavities. This will allow her eyes to sit back in a more natural position. She'll then have eye muscle surgery to realign them in an attempt to correct her diplopia. Afterwards, she'll need surgery for her eyelids. You can see pictures of Laura's before and after journey at her home page, *http://hometown.aol.com/ lisareynolds64/myhomepage/personal.html.*

The financial and emotional strain caused by her condition has been enormous. Laura was forced to resign from a job that she loved, and she no longer feels safe driving. She feels like a prisoner in her own home because her appearance deters her from socializing. She writes, "I am 38, but I look 58. This eye disease is worse than the thyroid disorder ever was for me. I feel like my life is on hold. I wouldn't wish this on anyone."

Laura wanted to share her story so that others would realize how important it is to take an active part in every aspect of their medical treatment. She also wants people to understand that, although there's still controversy surrounding the use of RAI, it really *does* affect the course of GO. Because RAI stimulates immune system cells within the thyroid gland, TSI (the antibodies responsible for congestive GO) continue to be produced. TSI are also released from dying thyroid cells. After RAI, TSI, levels rise, and can stay elevated for many years. Laura hopes that her story will educate and empower others.

Bill

My friend Bill, a middle-aged executive, was diagnosed with hypothyroidism at a routine physical in 1999. He was never told that his disorder was autoimmune. He was immediately prescribed 0.125 mg levothyroxine, and told to return in one year. He was told he would lead a normal life. At an office visit in 2000, his TSH was 2.80 mu/L (a normal range is 0.4-5.0 mu/L). Because he had begun to experience symptoms of hyperthyroidism, he started scheduling quarterly appointments. He soon realized that his TSH level was hardly stable. His TSH level was .06 mu/L on December 20th, 2000, and 3.05 mu/L in February 2001. And in December of 2001, his TSH was .01 mu/L—indicating that he was hyperthyroid. His TSH level has stayed suppressed ever since.

Bill's Eye Disease

In March 2002, Bill's doctor finally lowered his levothyroxine dose to 0.075 mg. About that time, Bill began experiencing diplopia. The previous September he'd noted extreme sensitivity to light, excessive tearing and swelling around his right eye. At the time, Bill had consulted three different doctors about his eye condition, including one at a renowned clinic. Not one of them mentioned that it could be thyroid-related. When he asked if there could possibly be a relationship between his eye symptoms and his thyroid disorder, they all scoffed at the question.

A new doctor Bill consulted when he moved to Hawaii immediately recognized his condition as GO, but recommended that Bill stay on the .075 mcg levothyroxine despite having a TSH of .01. This doctor also mentioned that there were other conditions that resembled GO, and ordered a CT scan and tests for thyroid and acetylcholine receptor antibodies.

Confirming GO

An orbital CT scan using contrast dye was performed in August 2002 to help determine the cause of Bill's diplopia. The orders indicated the diagnosis was thyroid orbitopathy or an orbital mass. The report read as follows.

> Findings: CT Scan of the orbits was performed in the axial plane at 1.3 mm intervals after the administration of 100 cc of Hypaque contrast material. This reveals thickening of the orbital musculature bilaterally, right greater than left. There is a bulbous configuration to the belly of the rectus muscles consistent with thyroid ophthalmopathy. The optic nerve is normal in caliber bilaterally. Both globes appear intact although proptotic.
>
> Impression: Findings consistent with thyroid ophthalmopathy. No intraconal masses are identified. No osseous abnormality is seen.

Bill's positive TSI results confirmed GO, and his negative results for acetylcholine receptor antibodies ruled out myasthenia gravis. Bill's doctor prescribed a short course of steroids (100 mg Prednisone for five days; 80 mg for four days; 60 mg for three days; 40 mg for two days; and 20mg for one day). Prednisone therapy offered no benefits for his eyes, although he reports noticing improvement in his knees, which had been pummeled during college by a number of sports injuries.

Resolution

After researching his condition on the Internet, and also asking my opinion, Bill realized that his hypothyroidism may have changed to hyperthyroidism. And excessive thyroid hormone could be contributing to his symptoms. He quit taking the levothyroxine in August of 2002. His TSH continued to be .01 mu/L in September, although his doctor is of the opinion that Bill is still hypothyroid. Bill's symptoms are now stabilizing and his ophthalmologist reports that Bill can have surgery to correct the diplopia after showing no signs of eye disease activity for six months.

Bill's Self-Care Protocol

Bill has also been experimenting—using aspirin to reduce his inflammation. He uses two tablets containing 325 mg of aspirin, and this appears to reduce symptoms of inflammation for up to three days. Bill also recommends using an eye patch to correct the diplopia. And, he's beginning to do eye exercises to help tone his eye muscles.

Bill has also noticed that salt aggravates his condition. He specifically notices an increase in swelling the morning after eating Italian and/or Mexican foods. And, Bill has experienced improvement after avoiding iodine in amounts greater than 150 mcg daily. He's found no effective relief for his light sensitivity, however. Consequently, he avoids sunlight and seeks out cloudy days. He also reports that in the early stages of GO, taping his eyes shut at night (using two pieces of tape applied horizontally) offered immediate relief. As the condition begins to stabilize, he reports, eye-taping is not as important.

Most importantly, Bill recommends that people verify everything a doctor tells them. Bill's first doctor insisted that once a patient becomes hypothyroid, he or she would always be hypothyroid. Bill has since learned that autoimmune thyroid disorders frequently change disposition depending on the autoantibodies predominating at a given time. Now he's aware that, because he has TSI antibodies, he could have either Hashitoxicosis or Graves' disease.

Bill also reminds those who are depressed about having GO that a tour of a local cancer hospital can really change one's outlook. Bill's been helped by Internet resources and online friends, and in an effort to give back some of what he's been given, he invites people who find themselves in similar situations to write to him at: *Bill711ana@aol.com*.

Mona

My friend Mona, a computer specialist in her early forties who lives in California, was diagnosed with Graves' disease in the summer of 1996. By autumn, she began noticing symptoms of thyroid eye disease, including a significant increase in floaters. She also experienced intermittent symptoms of eyelid retraction. These flare-ups would last for several weeks and then subside.

Treating Graves' disease

The first endocrinologist she consulted put her on a hefty dose of the anti-thyroid drug methimazole. After a few weeks, she developed an allergic reaction and was switched to the anti-thyroid drug PTU. Her doctor said she'd likely be intolerant of PTU (although people intolerant of one ATD generally have no trouble with other ATDs).

Mona tolerated PTU well however, and decided to find a doctor with more experience treating hyperthyroidism with medications. Unfortunately, the second doctor thought her good response to PTU was an indication of remission and discontinued it. Within five months, she developed migraine headaches, proptosis, dry eye, light sensitivity, and eye spasm, and her eyes constantly hurt. A measurement of her eye pressure showed that it had increased. She began using analgesics to help with the pain.

The Fear Factor

Thinking that her Graves' disease was cured, Mona feared that she'd developed a totally unrelated eye condition. She consulted an internist who tested her thyroid hormone levels. He called two days later and reported that she was extremely hyperthyroid.

When she subsequently called her endocrinologist, he suggested that her levels were merely high/normal, and he told her that she was depressed. She disagreed, and he reluctantly prescribed PTU. Within 48 hours her eye symptoms had improved.

Time for a Change

Mona began researching her condition on the Internet, and consulted a third endocrinologist. He was amused by her attempts to learn about her condition and promptly prescribed a dose of PTU that made her hypothyroid. Her symptoms of GO persisted. At this time she continued to see an ophthalmologist, and learned that he was very concerned about her increased eye pressure.

But Mona became irritated with the condescending attitude of her third endocrinologist. Through an Internet acquaintance, Mona met her fourth endocrinologist. This doctor stressed the importance of changing ATD doses gradually. As Mona's thyroid levels stabilized, her doctor decreased her dosage slowly. At one point in the course of weaning her off the PTU, he had her taking just a quarter of the smallest available tablet daily. She has now been in remission and off medications for nearly two years.

Improvement at Last

As Mona's thyroid condition improved, her proptosis and her eye pressure both decreased, showing that her GO was responding well to the treatment for her hyperthyroidism. In most cases, patients will notice improvement in their GO as their thyroid levels improve. And for most patients, this is the only treatment needed.

Mona still notices occasional floaters and discomfort, but she's convinced that her eye condition will continue to improve the longer she's in remission. She's noticed that both her thyroid levels and her eye symptoms worsen in times of stress.

Mona has also changed her diet—reducing her consumption of soda, sodium, chocolate, alcohol, spicy foods, fish and red meat. She's eating more vegetables and fruit, and drinking more water and fruit juices. She's also practicing stress reduction techniques.

Lately, she's eased up on some of her complementary therapies, but she continues to schedule regular appointments with both her endocrinologist and her ophthalmologist. She has routine blood thyroid function tests every few months, and makes sure that her levels stay within the normal range. After all that she's learned, Mona's made up her mind that if she happens to have a relapse—becoming hyperthyroid again—she'll use ATDs again. After the eye problems she's experienced, she's opposed to the idea of ever having radioiodine ablation to correct a future condition of hyperthyroidism.

Mary B

My friend Mary, a college professor and new mother in her mid-thirties, developed a sinus infection in January 1999 that lasted a good six to eight weeks. She consulted a doctor early on and took antibiotics for the duration of her infection. About this time, she began to experience eye pain. She attributed this to having a sinus infection. The eye pain persisted into March, although her sinus infection had cleared up. In addition, her eyes became scratchy, dry and uncomfortable.

Diagnosing Graves' Disease

In April, Mary began to feel out of sorts, and her eye problems persisted. She consulted a doctor who noticed that her eyes and thyroid gland were both protruding. The doctor ordered lab tests and confirmed that Mary was hyperthyroid.

The endocrinologist Mary consulted noted that her eye involvement was routine for Grave's disease. It was her opinion that Mary didn't need to see an ophthalmologist. Mary decided to consult one anyway. After researching doctors in her area, she realized that everyone she'd asked recommended the same ophthalmologist, a doctor on staff at a major research university.

Diagnosing GO

This ophthalmologist determined that Mary had moderately severe eye involvement. He noted that she didn't have exophthalmos, but she did have eyelid retraction that made her eyes appear prominent.

After doing a little research at an online Graves' disease support group, Mary began to use Refresh eye drops and started taping her eyes shut at night. She also invested in some attractive hats and eyeglasses to draw attention away from her appearance. Unable to wear her customary contact lenses, Mary had to get used to wearing prescription lenses again.

Mary's vision began to fluctuate dramatically. On some days she would see better out of one eye and on other days, the opposite. A CT scan showed that despite her blurred vision, she had no danger of optic nerve involvement. Mary believes that the moisture drops she was using may also have contributed to her inability to see clearly during this time.

Deciding on Therapy

Mary was initially prescribed the anti-thyroid drug propylthiouracil (PTU) to reduce her thyroid hormone levels. However, her liver enzyme levels began to rise, and she was unable to continue using PTU. Told she wasn't a candidate for ATDs, Mary considered having thyroidectomy surgery and consulted a surgeon. She scheduled surgery but decided to try using complementary therapies in the meantime.

Her complementary therpaies protocol included homeopathy, naturopathy, acupuncture, a macrobiotic diet and nutritional supplements. An herbalist recommended using the herb milk thistle, which is used to treat liver problems, as a therapy for her eye problems. During this time, Mary also stopped nursing her daughter, who had just turned one. Within three months of weaning her daughter and following her own holistic healing plan, Mary's hyperthyroidism went into remission.

Remission

By October of 1999, Mary no longer had to tape her eyes shut at night. She noted a dramatic improvement in her eyes, although she still was unable to wear contact lenses on a daily basis. And despite her improvement, her eyes remained dry.

Twenty percent of patients with Graves' disease spontaneously become hypothyroid as their immune systems begin to predominantly produce thyroglobulin and blocking TSH receptor antibodies. Mary became hypothyroid in 2001. At this time her eye problems began to flare and she developed extreme light sensitivity. Although she is now on thyroid replacement hormone to correct her hypothyroidism, her eye symptoms resurface whenever her TSH level rises above 2.0 mu/L. In January 2003, the American Association of Clinical Endocrinologists issued a press release, recommending that labs lower the reference range for TSH. The recommended range for patients on replacement hormone is 0.4-1.0 mu/L.

In 2001, Mary had eyelid surgery to correct the swelling and eyelid retraction caused by Graves' ophthalmopathy. She's satisfied with the results and recommends surgery for anyone unhappy with changes caused by GO. Although her insurance initially turned her down, they consented to pay for the procedure after seeing pictures of her before and after developing Graves' ophthalmopathy.

RESOURCES

National Organizations

American Academy of Ophthalmology
655 Beach Street
San Francisco, CA 94109
Tel: (415) 561-8500
Fax: (415) 561-8567
www.eyenet.org

American Association of Clinical Endocrinology
1000 Riverside Ave.
Jacksonville, FL 32204
Tel: (904) 353-7878
www.aace.com

American Foundation of Thyroid Patients
18634 North Lyford Dr.
Katy, TX 77449
Tel: (281) 855-6608
www.thyroidfoundation.org

American Thyroid Association
Montefiore Medical Center
111 East 210th Street
Bronx, NY 10467
www.ata.org

The National Eye Institute
National Eye Health Education Program
2020 Vision Place
Bethesda, MD 20892
Tel: (301) 496-5248
www.nei.nih.gov

National Center for Complementary and Alternative Medicine (NCCAM)
P.O. BOX 8218
Silver Spring, MD 20907-8218
Tel: (888) 644-6226
http://nccam.nih.gov

National Graves Disease Foundation
P.O. Box 1969
Brevard, NC 28712
www.ngdf.org

International Society for Orbital Disorders (ISOD)
Members of the society, in both Canada and the United States, are specialists in the treatment of thyroid related eye disorders. The following websites contain listings of current members.

Canadian Ophthalmologists
www.isod.net/Canada.html

United States Ophthalmologists
www.isod.net/USA.html

TED Head Office
Solstice, Sea Road
Winchelsea Beach, East Sussex TN36 4LH
United Kingdom
Tel/Fax: 01797-222-338
Email: *tedassn@eclipse.co.uk*

Ophthalmology Clinics Specializing in Thyroid Associated Eye Disorders

Kentucky Eye Institute
http://kyeye.com/institute

Eric Purdy, M.D.
Caylor-Nickel Clinic
Bluffton, Indiana 46714
Tel: (260) 824-3500

State Listings for Ophthalmology Referrals
American Foundation of Thyroid Patients, Ophthalmology Referrals
(Kelly Hale has created a list of ophthalmologists by state who are specifically trained
to diagnose and treat thyroid associated eye disease.)
www.thyroidfoundation.org/aftpopthalm3.html

Orthoptics Resources

International Orthoptics Association (IOA)
United States Branch
Department of Ophthalmology
Children's Hospital of New Orleans
200 Henry Clay Ave.
New Orleans, LA 70118
Contact: Cindy Pritchard
Tel: (504) 896-9426

American Orthoptic Council
3914 Nakoma Road
Madison, WI 53705
Tel: (608) 233-5383

American Orthoptic Journal
American Association of Certified Orthoptists
University of Wisconsin
www.aoj.org

Internet Resources

About.com Thyroid (hosted by Mary Shomon)
www.thyroid.about.com

American Foundation of Thyroid Patients
www.thyroidfoundation.org

Agency for Healthcare Research and Quality
www.ahrq.gov

Center for Disease Control (CDC)
www.cdc.gov

Daisy's Educational Graves' Disease Site
http://daisyelaine_co.tripod.com/gravesdisease/

Emedicine
www.emedicine.com/oph/

Exophthalmos Images in Endocrinology-Med Students
www.medstudents.com.br

Geocities Ocular Times
www.geocities.com/ocular_times/

Healthfinder
www.healthinder.gov

National Eye Institute
www.nei.nih.gov

National Library of Medicine (NLM)
www.nlm.nih.gov

National Library Service for the Blind and Handicapped
www.loc.gov/nls

Office of Rare Diseases

http://rarediseases.info.nih.gov/ord

Society for Endocrinology
www.endocrinology.org

St. Luke's Clinic
www.stlukeseye.com

Thyroid Manager Online Textbook
www.thyroidmanager.org/thyroidbook.htm

Thyroid Society for Education and Research
www.the-thyroid-society.org

University of Iowa Eye Center
http://webeye.ophth.uiowa.edu/

Journals

Archives of Ophthalmology
http://archopht.ama-assn.org/

British Journal of Ophthalmology
http://bjo.bmjjournals.com

Journal of Clinical Endocrinology & Metabolism
http://jcem.endojournals.org

Society of the European Journal of Endocrinology
www.eje.org

National Library of Medicine
Pub Med
www.ncbi.nlm.nih.gov/entrez/

Books

Kahaly, George, Ed. "Endocrine Ophthalmopathy: Molecular, Immunological and Clinical Aspects," *Developments in Ophthalmology*,

Thyroid Eye Disease

Vol 25.(Basel, Switzerland, S. Karger Publishing: 1993.)

Moore, Elaine A. *Graves' Disease, A Practical Guide*. (Jefferson, NC, McFarland Publishing: 2001.)

Pickardt, C. Renate and Boergen, Klaus Peter, Ed. *Graves' Ophthalmopathy: Developments in Diagnostic Methods and Therapeutical Procedures* (Developments in Ophthalmology, Vol 20). (Basel, Switzerland, S. Karger Publishing: 1989.)

Prummel, Mark F. *Recent Developments in Graves' Ophthalmopathy*. (The Netherlands, Kluwer Academic Publishers: 1994.)

Braverman, Lewis E. and Robert D. Utiger. *Werner and Ingbar's The Thyroid: A Fundamental and Clinical Text*, 8th ed. (Philadelphia, Lippincott Williams & Wilkins: 2000.)

Wall, Jack and How, Jacques, Ed. "Graves' Ophthalmopathy," *Current Issues in Endocrinology and Metabolism*. (London, Blackwell Science Inc.: 1990.)

GLOSSARY

Abductor muscle: The abductor muscles operate to turn the eye outward.

Acetylcholine receptor antibodies: Autoantibodies typically seen in myasthenia gravis; these antibodies block acetylcholine from triggering impulses and interfere with muscle contraction.

Adductor muscles: The adductor muscles operate to turn the eye inward.

Adenxa: The anatomical structures that protect and move the eyeball, such as eyelids and extraocular muscles.

Adrenergic: A chemical with physiologic effects similar to those of epinephrine; sympathomimetic.

Anterior chamber: The front half of the anterior compartment of the eyeball; this is the area between the cornea and iris.

Antibody: An immunoglobulin produced by the immune system's B lymphocytes after antigenic stimulation; antibodies are capable of reacting with the antigen that caused their production.

Antigen: A substance, usually a protein or lipid particle, capable of triggering an immune response.

Antithyroid drug (ATD): A drug used to block iodine absorption, interfering with thyroid hormone production; ATDs also have a mild immunosuppressant effect.

Thyroid Eye Disease

Astigmatism: A condition in which the uneven curvature of the cornea blurs and distorts both distant and near objects. An astigmatic eye has two different meridians, at 90 degrees to each other, which causes images to focus in different planes for each meridian. Astigmatism causes images to be out of focus no matter what the distance.

Autoantibody: An antibody directed at self components, such as orbital tissue cells, in thyroid eye disease.

Autoimmune disease: A disease that originates in the immune system, causing immune system cells to target self components. Autoimmune diseases may be organ-specific, targeting specific organs, or they may be systemic, targeting cells in various bodily organs.

Autoimmune thyroid disease (AITD): Any of a number of thyroid disorders, such as Graves' disease, which have an autoimmune origin.

B lymphocyte cell: A type of white blood cell involved in antibody production.

Beta blockers (beta adrenergic blocking agents): Medications, such as propranolol, that are used to block the adrenergic response.

Bhlepharoptosis: The drooping of an upper eyelid due to paralysis; ptosis.

Blepharoplasty: A type of eyelid surgery used to reduce droopy eyelids or eyebrows and "bags" under the eyes.

Blocking TSH receptor antibodies (Blocking TRAb): One of the subtypes of TSH receptor antibodies associated with hypothyroidism and the development of GO.

Chemosis: Edema of the bulbar conjunctiva that typically causes corneal swelling.

Choroid: The part of the middle or vascular layer of the eyeball; the choroid is attached to the inner surface of the "white of the eye" or sclera.

Ciliary body: The raised part of the middle or vascular layer of the eyeball that surrounds the lens and is attached to the lens by zonular fibers. The ciliary muscles control the shape of the lens.

Computed tomography scanning (CT or CAT scan): Imaging technique in which X-rays are passed through the body at different angles and analyzed by a computer.

Conjunctiva: The mucous membrane that lines the inner surface of the eyelids and is continued over the front of the eyeball.

Cornea: The transparent part of the coat of the eyeball that covers the iris and pupil and admits light into the interior.

Corticosteroids: Natural steroid hormones, including glucocorticoids and mineralocorticoids, or synthetic drugs, such as prednisone, used to supplement natural hormones; corticosteroids suppress the immune system and help prevent inflammation.

Cytokines: Hormone-like messenger proteins, such as interferon, produced during the immune response, which regulate the intensity and duration of the immune response. Cytokines are thought to play a role in the development and perpetuation of GO.

Cytotoxic: Having the ability to attack and destroy cells.

Diplopia: Visual disturbance causing objects to appear double; double vision. Most patients with GO have binocular diplopia, meaning that the double vision can be corrected when one eye is covered.

EMO syndrome:A syndrome of exophthalmos, pretibial or localized myxedema and osteoarthropathy. Patients may show no signs of abnormal thyroid dysfunction. Osteoarthritis may occur as a form of digital clubbing; myxedema may occur in the skin covering the shoulders rather than the typical pretibial area.

Enophthalmos: A sinking of the eyeball inward into the orbital cavity.

Epinephrine: An adrenergic hormone secreted by the adrenal medulla in response to stress.

Thyroid Eye Disease

Euthyroid: Characterized by normal thyroid function tests.

Euthyroid Graves' disease: A condition characterized by thyroid eye disease with no past history or current evidence of thyroid dysfunction.

Exophoria: Latent strabismus in which the visual axes tend outward toward the temple.

Exophthalmos: Protrusion of the eyeball from the orbit; proptosis.

Extraocular: Adjacent but exterior to the eyeball.

Extraocular muscles: The six tiny muscles that surround the eye and control its movements. These muscles work together to produce smooth eye movements and to help keep the eyes aligned.

Extrathyroidal: Situated or occurring away from the thyroid gland.

Eye: The organ associated with sight. Consists of the eyeball and adenxa.

Eye motility problems: Abnormalities in restriction of the eyes, particularly restriction of upward gaze, which may progress to a limitation of horizontal eye movement.

Eyelid: Two folds of skin that cover the anterior surface of the eyeball. (The conjunctiva covers the inner surface of the eye.)

Eyelid retraction: The inward folding of the eyelid, which may affect the upper or lower lids of one or both eyes. Early in the course of the disease, lid retraction may be due to the exaggerated sympathetic nervous system response seen in hyperthyroidism; in later disease stages, retraction may be caused by fibrosis (scarring or the presence of collagen deposits).

Fibroadipose: Having both fibrous (dense, for instance scar tissue) and adipose (fatty) characteristics.

Fibroblast: An immature fibrous connective tissue cell that ultimately differentiates into either chrondoblasts, collagenoblasts, orbital tissue cells, and osteoblasts (bone cells).

Fibrosis: The process by which tissues changes texture, becoming fibrous or woody, with an appearance similar to scar tissue.

Free thyroxine or T4 (FT4): The unbound form of the thyroid hormone thyroxine that has been cleaved from binding protein and is available to react with the body's cells.

Free triiodothyronine or T3 (FT3): The unbound form of the thyroid hormone triiodothyronine that has been cleaved from binding protein and is available to react with the body's cells.

Fundoscopy: The study of the fundus by ophthalmology examination.

Fundus: The part of the eye opposite the pupil.

Glucocorticoid: Any of a class of steroid hormones that are produced by the adrenal cortex during stress, or synthetically (for instance, Prednisone). Glucorticoids inhibit the immune response and reduce inflammation.

Glycosaminoglycan (GAG): Any of a class of polysaccharides, for instance, hyaluronic acid, that form mucins when complexed with protein molecules. Increased amounts of GAG deposited into the orbital cavity contribute to the congestive infiltration of Graves' ophthalmopathy.

Goiter: An enlargement of the thyroid gland resulting from hypothyroidism, hyperthyroidism, or an inflammatory process.

Graves' disease: An autoimmune hyperthyroid disorder sometimes associated with a related dermal condition or the ophthalmologic condition known as Graves' ophthalmopathy.

Graves' ophthalmopathy (GO): An eye disease characterized by exophthalmos, blurring, dryness, diplopia, lid retraction, and other symptoms, which primarily occurs in people with autoimmune thyroid disease, although it may occur in individuals with no past history or current evidence of thyroid disease.

Grittiness: A condition of eye dryness in which the eyes feel as if they have sand in them.

Thyroid Eye Disease

Hashimoto's thyroiditis (HT): An autoimmune hypothyroid disorder associated with the development of GO.

Hashitoxicosis: Coexisting symptoms of hyperthyroidism in a patient with Hashimoto's thyroiditis.

Helper T lymphocyte: The subset of T lymphocytes bearing CD4, which scout for specific foreign antigens and play an instrumental role in the immune response.

Heterophoria: Latent strabismus in which one eye tends to deviate either medially or laterally.

Human leukocyte antigen (HLA): The antigenic marker for immune system genes of the major histocompatibility complex (MHC) occurring on the short arm of chromosome 6 in humans; specific HLA antigens regulate the immune response and confer susceptibility to different autoimmune conditions.

Hypertropia: An elevation of the line of vision of one eye above that of the other; upward strabismus.

Immune system: The network of cells, organs and chemicals that work together to protect the body from foreign substances and to destroy infected and malignant cells.

Immunoglobulin: A protein with several subtypes, which has properties of an antibody; antibody.

Immunomodulator: A substance capable of modulating, strengthening or balancing the immune system.

Immunosuppressive: Having the ability to inhibit or reduce immune system activity.

Inferior: Situated below and closer to the feet; situated in a more posterior or ventral position in the body.

Iodine: The organic form of iodine, which combines with the amino acid tyrosine to form thyroid hormone. As a dietary substance, iodine is known to influence the development of autoimmune thyroid disorders.

IOP: Intraocular pressure, the pressure within the eyeball that gives it its round shape.

Iris: The opaque muscular contractile diaphragm that is suspended in the aqueous humor in front of the lens of the eye, is perforated by the pupil and is continuous peripherally with the ciliary body of the eye. The iris has a deep pigmented posterior surface which excludes the entrance of light except through the pupil and a colored anterior surface which determines the color of the eyes.

Keratitis: Inflammation of the cornea.

Lacrimal apparatus: Consists of the lacrimal gland (which produces tears), the lacrimal puncta (two openings that collect lacrimal secretions into the lacrimal duct), and the lacrimal duct.

Lacrimation: The secretion of tears, especially excessive secretion.

Lagophthalamos: A condition of lid lag or incomplete eyelid closure.

Latent: Existing in hidden or dormant form.

Lateral: Lying at or extending toward the right or left side; lying away from the median axis of the body.

Lens: The solid, transparent structure separating the anterior compartment from the vitreous (posterior) compartment of the eyeball; the lens is attached to the ciliary body by the zonular fibers. The lens focuses transmitted objects onto the retina.

Limbus: The marginal region of the cornea of the eye by which it is continuous with the sclera.

Lymphoma: A tumor arising from any of the cellular elements of lymph nodes, particularly B lymphocytes.

Macrophage: A type of large white blood cell that engulfs or ingests foreign particles and infectious microorganisms by a process known as phagocytosis.

Magnetic resonance imaging (MRI): An imaging technique based on magnetic fields and low-energy radio waves with the ability to bypass bone and examine internal structures.

Medial: Lying or extending toward the middle axis of the body.

Methimazole: A type of antithyroid drug used in the United States; similar to the European drug carbimazole.

Myasthenia gravis: An autoimmune disorder characterized by impaired transmission of motor nerve impulses, causing episodic weakness and muscle fatigue.

Myopia: An eye condition in which parallel rays are focused in front of the retina, causing nearsightedness.

Myositis: Muscle inflammation.

Myxedema: A condition of mucin accumulation typically seen in hypothyroidism.

Nasolacrimal duct: The duct that collects lacrimal secretions from the conjunctival sac and transmits the collected tear solution into the ventral nasal meatus just posterior to the external nasal nares.

Neuropathy: Inflammation or injury directed against nerves.

Ocreotide: The somatostatin analog used in the treatment of GO.

Ocular injection: Congestion occurring in the orbital cavity.

Ophthalmologist: A doctor specializing in diseases of the eye.

Ophthalmopathy: Any disease affecting the eye or related orbital structures.

Ophthalmoplegi: Paralysis of eye muscles, particularly on upward gaze.

Optic disc: The white, raised area on the posterior surface of the vitreous compartment associated with the entrance of the optic nerve through the wall of the eyeball.

Optic nerve: The second cranial nerve that functions to transmit impulses from the retina to the brain, where they're interpreted as vision.

Optic neuropathy: A disorder or compression of the optic nerve, which may result in blindness.

Orbit: The bony socket that houses the eyeball.

Orbital apex: The back or rear portion of the orbital cavity.

Orbital decompression: The type of surgery used to reduce the congestive infiltration of GO.

Orbital fibroblasts: Immature orbital tissue cells, which, upon maturation, become orbital cells.

Orbital fissure: Either of two openings transmitting nerves and blood vessels to the orbit; one fissure is situated superiorly between the greater wing and the lesser wing of the sphenoid bone; the other is situated inferiorly between the greater wing of the sphenoid bone and the maxilla.

Palpebral fissure: The space between the margins of the eyelids.

Photobia: Abnormal sensitivity or intolerance to light; light sensitivity.

Plasmapheresis: The procedure in which phlebotomy is performed and the blood cells returned to the donor, thereby reducing the plasma concentration in an attempt to lower antibody levels.

Proptosis: A protrusion of the eyeball; exophthalmos.

Psychoneuroimmunology (PNI): The study of the intricate relationship between the immune, nervous and endocrine systems.

Ptosis: An eyelid problem caused by paralysis of the third nerve or from sympathetic innervation, which allows the upper eyelids to droop.

Pupil: The opening formed by the iris that controls the amount of light that enters the vitreous compartment of the eyeball.

Radioiodine: Any of nine radioisotopes of iodine used in diagnostic studies and ablative treatment.

Radioiodine ablation: The therapeutic destruction of thyroid cells by the radioiodine isomer I-131 in an attempt to reduce the amount of functional thyroid cells capable of producing thyroid hormone.

Radiotherapy: The medical use of external beam irradiation. Orbital radiotherapy is used as a treatment in GO.

Retina: The inner or nervous layer of the eyeball; the retina is responsible for transmitting visual signals as electrical impulses to the brain via the central nervous system.

Retrobulbar: Pertaining to the area behind the orbital cavity.

Sagittal: Shaped like or resembling an arrow; straight; referring to an anteroposterior plane or section parallel to the median plane of the body.

Sclera: Dense, white, opaque fibrous coat enclosing the eyeball except for the part covered by the cornea; commonly referred to as the "whites of the eyes."

Septum: The dividing wall or membrane, especially between bodily spaces or masses of soft tissue.

Somatostatin: A polypeptide hormone produced in the brain and pancreas.

Sphenoid bone: The compound bone situated at the base of the cranium, which is formed by the fusion of several bony elements; the sphenoid bone consists of a median body with lateral extensions that form a pair of great wing-like expansions; the front portion of the sphenoid bone also has a pair of lateral triangular-shaped extensions and two large ventral processes that extend downward toward the orbital cavity.

Sphincter pupillae: The broad flat band of smooth muscle in the iris that surrounds the pupil of the eye.

Strabismus: An ophthalmic condition characterized by an inability of the eyes to focus together as a consequence of a defect in one or more eye muscles. Strabismus may cause the eyes to roll upward or downward in their sockets, or they may not move together laterally, obscuring vision and causing squinting or diplopia.

Subclinical: Pertaining to an early stage of a disease in which there may be no clinical symptoms.

Superior: Toward the head and away from the feet; situated in a more anterior or dorsal position in the body.

Suppressor T lymphocytes: The subset of T cells able to inhibit T cell or B cell reactivity, preventing the autoimmune response.

Sympathomimetic: Mimicking stimulation of the sympathetic nervous system.

Thyroid stimulating hormone (TSH): The pituitary hormone that helps to regulate thyroid hormone levels' thyrotropin.

Thyroid stimulating hormone (TSH, thyrotropin) receptor antibodies (TRAb): Autoantibodies to the TSH receptor, responsible for autoimmune thyroid disorders. TRAb include stimulating (TSI), blocking and binding (TBII) antibodies.

Thyroid stimulating immunoglobulins (TSI): Stimulating TSH receptor antibodies, which cause symptoms of hyperthyroidism in Graves disease. TSI are also known to activate orbital fibroblasts, contributing to the development of GO.

Thyroxine (T4): The major thyroid hormone consisting of 4 iodine atoms. Considered a prohormone, the majority of T4 is converted to the more potent triiodothyronine (T3) in the body.

Traditional Chinese Medicine (TCM): A medical discipline based on historical Chinese healing philosophies; TCM includes acupuncture, herbal medicine, acupressure and diet.

Triiodothyronine (T3): The thyroid hormone produced by the thyroid gland as well as by peripheral (away from the thyroid gland) conversion from T4; approximately 5 to 10 times more potent than T4.

Tyrosine: An amino acid that combines with iodine to form thyroid hormone and its iodothyronine precursors.

Ultrasonography (Ultrasound): A diagnostic imaging technique utilizing reflected ultrasonic waves to delineate, measure and examine internal body structures or organs based on changes in tissue density.

Uvea: The vascular layer of the eyeball, consisting of the choroids, ciliary body, and iris.

Visual acuity: How sharply or clearly a person can see at a distance.

Visual field exam: Assesses the total area where objects can be seen in the peripheral vision while the eye is focused on a central point.

Vitreous fluid: A jelly-like fluid found within the vitreous compartment of the eyeball, which is the internal compartment of the eyeball bounded by the lens and retina.

Zonular fibers: Fibers that attach the edge of the lens to the ciliary body.

BIBLIOGRAPHY

Bartalena, Luigi, Marcocci, Claudio, et al., "Cigarette Smoking and Treatment Outcomes in Graves' Ophthalmopathy," *Annals of Internal Medicine*, Brief Communications, Oct 98.

Binaghi, M., Levy, C., Douvin, C. et al., "Severe thyroid ophthalmopathy related to interferon alpha therapy," *J Fr Ophtalmol*, April, 2002; 25(4): 412-415.

Bouzas, E., Karadimas, P., et al., "Antioxidant agents in the treatment of Graves' ophthalmopathy," *American Journal of Ophthalmopathy*, 2000 May; 129(5): 618-622.

Burch, Henry, et al., "Ophthalmopathy," in *Werner & Ingbar's The Thyroid, A Fundamental and Clinical Text*, 8th Edition, Lewis Braverman and Robert Utiger, Editors. (Philadelphia, Lippincott Williams & Wilkins, 2000, 531.)

Chiovatoe, L., et al., "Outcome of Thyroid Function in Graves' Patients Treated with Radioiodine: Role of Thyroid Stimulating and Thyrotropin Blocking Antibodies and of Radioiodine Induced Thyroid Damage," *Journal of Clinical Endocrinology and Metabolism*, 83(1): 40-46.

DeGroot, Leslie, et al., "Complications in Graves' Disease, Thyroid Disease Manager," *The Thyroid and its Diseases*, Chap 12, updated Sept, 2002, via the internet, *www.thyroidmanager.org/thyroidbook.htm*

Frewin, S., Dickinson, A., et al., "Self-consciousness, psychological and social functioning in thyroid eye disease," *TED*, a publication of the

Thyroid Disease Association, 2000, Mar, issue 49.

Gerding, M.N., van der Meer, J., et al., "Association of thyrotropin receptor antibodies with the clinical features of Graves' ophthalmopathy," *Clinical Endocrinology*, 2000 Mar; 52(3):267-271.

Goldberg, R.A., Kim A.J., Kerivan, K.M., "The lacrimal keyhole, orbital door jamb, and basin of the inferior orbital fissure. Three areas of deep bone in the lateral orbit." *Archives of Ophthalmology*, 1998 Dec; 116(12): 1618-1624.

Gorman, C., "Radiotherapy for Graves' Ophthalmopathy: Results at One Year," *Thyroid*, 2002 Mar;12(3):251-255.

Kahaly, G., Hardt, J., Petrak, F. and U. Egle, "Psychosocial factors in subjects with thyroid-associated ophthalmopathy," *Thyroid*, 2002 Mar; 12(3): 237-239.

Kazim, Michael, Trokel, Stephen, Acaroglu, Golge and Alexandra Elliott, "Reversal of dysthyroid optic neuropathy following orbital fat decompression," *British Journal of Ophthalmology Online* 2000, June; 84: 600-605.

Kim, W., Chung, H., et al., "Clinical significance of classification of Graves' disease according to the characteristics of TSH receptor antibodies," *Korean Journal of Internal Medicine*, 2001, Sept; 16(3): 187-200.

Kinyoun, J., et al., "Radiation therapy for Graves' ophthalmopathy," *Archives of Ophthalmology*, 1984;102: 1473.

Korinth, M.C., et al., "Follow-up of extended pterional orbital decompression in severe Graves' ophthalmopathy," *Acta Neurochir,* 2002 Feb; 144(2): 113-120.

Liao, S., Huang, Y., and L. Li, "Clinical observation on treatment of thyrotoxic exophthalmos with jiayanxiao plus Tapazole," Abstract, via PubMed, the Internet.

Life Extension Staff, "The Aging Eye," *Life Extension*, Feb 2002, 36-41.

Lisai, S., Marino, M., Pinchera, A., et al., "Thyroglobulin in orbital tissues from patients with thyroid-associated ophthalmopathy: predominant localization in fibroadipose tissue," *Thyroid*, 2002 May; 12(5): 351-360.

Marquez, S.D., et al., "Long-term results of irradiation for patients with progressive Graves' ophthalmopathy, *Int Radiat Oncol Biol Phys*, 2001, Nov 1;51(3): 766-777.

Mondoa, Emil, M.D. and Mindy Kitei, *Sugars That Heal*. (New York, Ballantine: 2001.)

Mourits, M., Koorneef, L., et al. "Clinical criteria for the assessment of disease activity in Graves' ophthalmopathy: a novel approach," *British Journal of Ophthalmology*, 1989; 73:639-644.

Noth, D., et al., "Graves' ophthalmopathy: natural history and treatment outcomes," *Swiss Med Wkly*, 2001; 131 (41-42), 603.

Perros, P., Kendall-Taylor, P., Crombie, A., "Natural history of thyroid associated ophthalmopathy," *Clinical Endocrinology*, 1995; 42-45.

Prummel, M.F., et al., "Randomised double-blind trial of prednisone vs radiotherapy in Graves' ophthalmopathy," *Lancet*, 1995; 342L949-954.

Salvi, M., Dazzi, D., et al., "Classification and prediction of the progression of thyroid-associated ophthalmopathy by an artificial neural network," *Ophthalmology*, 2002 Sep;109(9): 1703-1708.

Smith, J.R. and J.T .Rosenbaum, "A role for methotrexate in the management of non-infectious orbital inflammatory disease," *Br J Ophthalmol*, 2001 Oct; 85(10):1220-1224.

Terwee, C., Dekker, F., Mourits, M., et al., "Interpretation and validity of changes in scores on the Graves' ophthalmopathy quality of life questionnaire (GO-QOL) after different treatments," *Clinical Endocrinology*, 2001, Mar; 54(3): 391-398.

Tong, N., Xiao, Y., Huang, H., and S. Wei, "A pair-matched comparison and follow-up study of patients with euthyroid GO and patients with hyperthyroid GO," *The Journal of Clinical Endocrinology and Metabolism*, 2002, 87(8): 3853.

Vaidya, B., Imrie, H., et al., "Cytotoxic T lymphocyte antigen 4 (CTLa-4) gene polymorphism confers susceptibility to thyroid associated orbitopathy," *Lancet*, Aug 99,354(9180); 743-745.

Walsh, John, "Radioiodine and thyroid eye disease," *British Medical Journal*, 1999, July, Issue 7202: 68-70.

Watkins, Lynnette, *Graves' Ophthalmopathy*, Department of Ophthalmology & Visual Sciences, University of Iowa, 1999, online *http://webeye.ophth.uiowa.edu/dept/DIAGTRT/Graves/graves.htm*.

Wessels, Izak, "Diplopia," Emedicine via the Internet, *www.emedicine.com/oph/topic191.htm*.

Wiersinga, W. M. and M. F. Prummel, "Pathogenesis of Graves' Ophthalmopathy—Current Understanding," *The Journal of Clinical Endocrinology and Metabolism*, 86(5): 502.

Yeatts, Patrick, M.D., "Graves' Ophthalmopathy," in *Endocrine Emergencies*, Volume 79 of *The Medical Clinics of North America*, Philadelphia, W.B. Saunders, 1995, 201.

INDEX

Abadie's sign 32
Abduction 52-53
Ablative treatment (thyroid) 28, 77-79, 141-143, 147-148
Acetylcholine receptor antibodies 99
Aching 44, 60
Active phase of GO 22, 30, 44, 66, 81-82, 103-104, 109, 123
Adduction 52-53
Adhesion molecules 80
Adhesions 123
Adipocytes 64, 66, 73
Age 76-77
Allergens 81, 130, 133, 142
American Thyroid Association 45
Amphetamines 81
Anatomy (eye) 49-61
Antibodies 64-65, 67-69
Antidepressant medications 57, 81, 108
Antigens 68, 80, 133
Antihistamines 57, 81, 96
Antioxidant vitamins 129-130
Antithyroid drugs (ATDs) 79, 102, 113-114, 142-143, 152-155
Appearance 18, 28, 38-39, 102, 104, 117, 139
Aqueous humor 32, 54
Artificial neural network 47
Artificial tears 60, 106-108
Astigmatism 33, 39
Asymmetrical eye disease 21, 38
Autoantibodies 64, 69-70, 133
Autoimmune disorders 12, 16, 43, 76, 133

Autoimmune form of GO 16, 67-73, 75, 118
Autoimmune thyroid disease 11-12, 27, 64, 67, 78, 83, 98
Autoreactive cells 69, 133
Ballet's sign 32
Bee pollen 135
Bejing Medical University 40
Beta adrenergic blocking agents 28, 102, 108
Bilateral eye retraction 38, 83
Bilateral proptosis 21, 97
Bilateral symmetry 21, 31, 40, 61
Binocular diplopia 22, 90-91
Binocular vision 22, 59, 116
Blepharoplasty 126
Blind spot 32, 56
Blindness- see Visual loss
Blinking 31-32, 60
Blocking TSH receptor antibodies 20, 64-65, 72-73
Blood vessels 17, 55
Blurred vision 18, 21, 29, 33-34, 39, 59-60, 85, 99
Boston's sign 33
Botox 127
Bowman's layer 55
Brain 50-52, 56, 96
Bromocriptine 127
Canthorrhapy 125
Canthus 57, 120
Cataracts 110, 116
Categories of GO 43, 45, 102
Catecholamines 28, 106

Cellular changes 63-66
Cerebrospinal fluid 98
Chemicals 78
Chemosis 34, 46, 60
Children 77
Choroidal folds 38, 88
Choroid 32, 50, 92
Cigarette smoke 13, 20, 75, 79-80, 129, 140
Ciliary body 32, 51
Circulation (eye) 28
City Hess Screen 88
Classifications of GO 45-48, 85
Clinical activity score 46-47, 65
Cocaine 81
"Coke bottle" eye muscle changes 91-92
Colcichine 111
Collagen 35, 55, 59, 66, 70
Collagen stimulating immunoglobulins (CSI) 85
Color desaturation 23-24
Color vision 18, 23-24, 34, 36, 47, 85-86
Commisurres 120
Complementary therapy 129-137
Computed tomography (CT) 19, 47, 91-92, 94-95, 97, 150-151
Cones 50-52
Congestion (orbital) 20, 36, 44, 48, 59, 115-116
Congestive infiltration 21, 25, 27, 40, 43, 57-59, 63-65, 103, 131
Conjunctiva 16, 32, 34, 37, 45, 57, 89
Conjunctival exposure 34,
Conjunctival injection 60, 89
Connective tissue 16, 24, 50-52, 54
Contractures 45
Cornea 17, 32, 34-35, 38-39, 45-46, 50-51, 54-56, 60-61
Corneal exposure 34, 39, 45, 60-61
Corneal perforation 39, 102
Corneal ulceration 34-35, 38, 43, 60-61, 118, 125
Corrugator muscle 58
Corticosteroids 44, 59-60, 79
Cortisol 78

Cosmetic surgery 38, 117, 139
Cover test 88
Crohn's disease 73
CTL4 genes 76
Cushing's syndrome 96
Cyclosporine 110-111
Cytokines 18, 64-66, 70-73, 78, 110, 126
Dalrymple's sign 32
Decompression see Orbital decompression
Decongestants 57, 81
Dehydration 40, 57, 106
Depression (eye muscle) 53
Descemet's membrane 55
Diagnosis 43, 83-99
Diet 28, 43, 75-77, 80-81, 117, 130, 133
Diplopia 16-17, 22, 25, 31, 34, 39-40, 44-45, 47, 60, 85-86, 90-91, 102, 108, 111, 116-117, 123-126, 137
Disc 24, 56
Discomfort (orbital) 39, 60
Diuretics 106, 113
Double vision see Diplopia
Dry eye 38, 56-57, 81, 106, 129
Dry phase of GO 44-45
Dryness (eye) 16, 27, 31, 36, 38-39, 43, 45, 56-57, 60, 101
Dysthyroid ophthalmopathy 18
Edema 18, 34, 36-37, 40, 45-46, 57, 63, 66, 98
Elevation (eye muscle) 53
EMO syndrome 98
Endocrine ophthalmopathy 18
Endothelium 56, 63
Endocrine disruptors 78
Endocrine system 13, 132
Energy healing 136
Enroth's sign 33
Environmental factors 12-13, 29, 76-82
Epithelium 55, 60
Epitheliopathy 45, 60
Essential fatty acids 131
Estrogens 78
Ethmoid sinus 118, 120
Ethnic differences 58

Euthyroid 22, 28, 40-41, 85
Euthyroid Graves' disease 1, 19-20, 22, 28, 40-41
Exercise 82, 133
Exophoria 34
Exophthalmic ophthalmoplegia 61
Exophthalmometer 24, 34, 94
Exophthalmos 16, 24, 34, 45-46, 48, 61, 98, 140
Exposure keratitis 39, 59, 87
Extended pterional orbit decompression 121-122
External beam radiotherapy 22, 44, 103, 105, 114-116
Extorsion 53
Extraocular muscles 16-17, 19, 22-24, 30, 37, 39, 45, 47, 50-55, 59, 63, 66, 88, 91-92, 105, 111, 113
Extrathyroidal 29-30
Eye anatomy and physiology 49-61
Eye exercises 136-137
Eye muscle alignment 16, 22
Eye muscle see Extraocular muscles
Eye muscle enlargement 16-17, 29, 54, 57-58, 60, 63, 72
Eye muscle restriction 16-17, 35, 39, 46
Eye muscle surgery 117, 124-126
Eye patches 108
Eyeball 50-51
Eyelashes 51
Eyelid retraction 17, 23, 28, 32, 35, 39, 43, 60, 155
Eyelid signs 19, 32-33
Eyelid surgery 125-127
Eyelids 32-33,38-40, 44, 51, 89, 119, 126
Facial muscles 58, 119
Fatty tissue 16
Fibrosis 35, 37, 40, 44-45, 59-60, 63, 93, 115
Flaxseed oil 131
Floaters 152
Fluoroscein angiography 92
Focus 25, 51
Forced duction testing 91, 117
Foreign body sensation 36, 39, 57, 61

Fovea 32, 52
Free T3 (FT3) 22, 85
Free T4 (FT4) 22, 85
Fresnel prisms 108
Frontalis muscle 58
Fundus 24, 88
Gadolinium 93
Gallium 67, 93-94
Gaze 31, 39
Gellinek's sign 33
Genes 12, 75
Genetic factors 12, 29, 75-76
Gifford's sign 33
Glabelar muscles 127
Glaucoma, 89, 92, 96, 108
Globe 46, 48-49, 51, 58
Glyconutrients 81, 134-135
Glycosaminoglycan (GAG) 24, 29, 35, 54, 63, 66, 70-72, 89-90, 109, 112, 123
Goffroy's sign 33
Graves' disease 11, 15, 19, 28, 30, 65, 67, 70, 73, 76, 84, 97, 99, 132, 141, 147, 154
Graves' eye disease 19, 132
Griffith's sign 33
Grittiness 15-16, 31, 36, 39, 45, 56-57, 107
Hashimoto's thyroiditis 11, 19-20, 23, 65, 67, 70, 84, 147
Hashitoxicosis 20, 26, 67, 147
Headache 98, 126
Heat shock proteins 79
Herbal medicine 129, 131, 133
Hertel exophthalmometer 24, 47, 84, 88
Hess screen 47, 88
Heterophoria 36
HLA markers 63, 68, 71, 75-76
Hydrocephalus 96
Hypertropia 36
Hyperthyroidism 11, 15, 23, 25-26, 28, 35, 48, 77, 102, 105
Hypokalemic periodic paralysis 96
Hypothyroidism 1, 15, 19, 21, 25, 28, 65, 79, 141, 149, 156
Imaging studies 40, 57, 84, 91

Immune response 13, 66, 71, 75, 133
Immune system 13, 16-17, 63, 68, 75-76, 82, 132-133
Immune system cells 59, 68, 78
Immunoglobulins 63, 69, 81, 111
Immunomodulators 133-134
Immunosuppressant agents 103, 110-112
Inactive phase of GO 44-45
Inferior oblique muscle 53, 91, 122
Inferior rectus muscle 50, 53, 91, 125
Inflammation 16-17, 21, 25, 29, 35, 39-40, 44-45, 57-60, 96, 109, 129, 151
Inflammatory response 17-18
Insurance 126
Interferon 12, 66, 70, 81
Interleukin 12, 66, 70
Intorsion 54
Intraocular pressure 59, 96, 108
Intravenous immunoglobulins 110, 112
Iodine 12, 77-78
Iris 17, 32, 50
Joffroy's sign 33
Jolethin 132
Keratitis 34-35, 39, 60
Keratoconus 90
Keratopathy 43, 59-61, 107, 118
Knie's sign 33
Lacrimal glands 40, 49, 119, 122
Lacrimation see Tearing
Lagophthalmos 47, 60
Laser polarimetry 92
Lateral rectus muscle 53, 57, 91
Lens 17, 32, 50-52, 54
Levator muscle 23, 28, 32, 39, 119, 122
Levator palpebrae superioris 49
Lid fissure width 47, 88-89, 105
Lid lag 32, 36, 47, 60, 77, 89, 107
Lifestyle 13-14, 129
Ligaments (orbital) 51
Light sensitivity see Photophobia
Limbus 89
Lithium 96-97
Local protective measures 101, 106
Lower eyelid 28, 49, 125

Lymphocytes 63-65, 68-71, 103, 110, 123, 133
Lymphoma 97
Macula 17, 51-52, 86
Magnetic resonance imaging 19, 92-93
Malignant exophthalmos 61
Maxillary sinus 50, 118, 120
Means' sign 33
Medial rectus muscle 53
Meditation 82
Men 77
Metronidazole 127
Midfacial muscles 58
Monoclonal antibody therapy 73
Monocular diplopia 22, 90-91
Motility (eye muscle) 17, 23-25, 35, 39-40, 45-46
Mourits 46-47, 65
Muller's muscle 48, 106, 125
Muscles (eye) 16-17, 38, 50-55, 58, 60
Muscle bellies 57
Myasthenia gravis 32, 83, 91, 96-97, 99, 144
Myopathy 43, 77
Myopia 96
Myositis 57
Myxedema 28
Nervous system 13, 51
Neurophthalmologist 102-103
NOSPECS 45-46
Nystagmus 116
Oblique eye muscles 23, 52-55
Occlusive lenses 108
Ocreotide 110-111
Ocreotide scintigraphy 93-94
Ocular pressure 21
Oculomotor nerve 56
Ophthalmologist 15, 84
Ophthalmoplegia 31, 45, 61, 91, 102
Ophthalmoscopy 89
Optic canal 60
Optic nerve 17, 29, 31-32, 40, 50, 56, 89, 117
Optic nerve compression 31
Optic nerve damage 38, 60, 86, 88-89

Optic neuropathy 17, 21, 24, 31, 36, 38, 43, 45-46, 59-60, 85-86, 102, 109
Optic neuritis 98-99
Orbicularis oculi 50
Orbicularis muscle 58
Orbit 49-51
Orbital anatomy 49-61
Orbital apex 60, 118
Orbital axis 52
Orbital cavity 16, 24, 29, 50, 54
Orbital congestion 54-59
Orbital decompression 18, 24, 37, 60, 104, 117-124
Orbital edema 57
Orbital fat 16, 54, 58, 60, 121, 123-124
Orbital fat decompression 123-124
Orbital fat orbitotomy 121
Orbital fibroblast cells 63-65, 70-71
Orbital plate of frontal bone 40
Orbital radiotherapy see External beam radiotherapy
Orbital rim 58, 122
Orbital septum 120
Orbital volume 21, 54, 58
Orbital walls 118-121
Orthoptics 116-117
Osteoarthropathy 98
Pain (eye) 15, 18, 35-36, 46, 60, 104, 109, 154
Palpebral fissure 48, 57
Panophthalmitis 35
Parabulbar 16
Paralysis (eye muscle) 31-32, 59, 61, 91
Parks 3-Step Test 91
Pathology of GO 57-61
Pentoxyfylline 110, 112
Perimetry testing 87, 89, 96
Periorbital edema 27-28, 36, 39, 60
Peripheral vision 86-87, 89
Phases of GO 44-45
Photophobia 36, 38, 44, 47, 58, 60, 106
Pigment (eye) 50
Pigmentation (eyelid) 33
Plasmapheresis 106, 112-113
Plateau phase 44, 103
Pop-eyed 48

Postpartum thyroiditis 25
Preadipocytes 64
Pred-G drops 125
Prednisone see Corticosteroids
Pressure (eye) 16, 21, 59, 153
Pretibial myxedema 23, 98
Prevalence of GO 19-20
Prisms 108
Procerus muscle 58
Progression 45, 102
Progressive exophthalmos 61
Proptosis 16-17, 21, 24, 28-29, 34-36, 38-39, 46-48, 54, 58, 60, 81, 84, 96-97, 102, 118
Pseudotumor cerebri 98
Pseudotumors 32, 92, 97
Psychoneuroimmunology (PNI) 132
Psychosocial effects 38, 139-156
Ptosis 96, 123
Puffiness 33, 40, 57
Punctate lesions 45, 60
Pupil 17, 33, 51
Quality of life 139, 140
Radioiodine, ablative treatment 15, 21, 25, 73, 77-79, 113, 141-143, 147-148
Reading 51
Rectus inferior muscle 50
Rectus superior muscle 50
Redness 16-17, 39, 44, 46, 57, 107
Refraction 51-52, 87
Remission 14
Resolution phase 44-45
Retina 17, 32, 50-52, 54, 92
Retrobulbar 16, 109
Retrobulbar pressure 16
Retrobulbar tissue 66
Rheumatoid arthritis 57
Riboflavin 135-136
Riesman's sign 33
Rods 50-52
Rosenbach's sign 33
Rotation (eye muscle) 52-53
Saturated fats 75, 81
Scarring 28, 35, 37, 55
Scar tissue 37, 59

Sclera 17, 32, 50-51, 57
Scleral spacer 125
Self-care 130
Selye, Hans 123
Severity of GO 45, 85
Sex 77
Sex steroids 12
Sight 50
Signs 31-33, 38, 40, 45-47, 60
Single photon emission CT 93-95
Sinusitis 123
Sjogren's syndrome 57
Slit-lamp examinations 60, 87-89
Smoking *see* Cigarette smoke
Snellen chart 46, 86-87
Soft tissue changes 24, 45-47, 112
Soparkar, Charles 132
Spastic signs 31, 40, 48
Sphenoid 119
Squinting 25
Stages of GO 43, 103
Stare 16-17, 28, 38, 47, 146
Stellwag's sign 32
Steroid therapy *see* Corticosteroids
Stimulating TSH receptor antibodies 20,
       44, 63-65
STIR MRI 93
Strabismus 24-25, 34, 36-37, 59
Stress 12, 29, 43, 75, 78-79, 81-82
Stroma 55-56, 60
Suborbicularis fat 58
Subtypes of GO 27-30
Sugar 13, 75, 80
Superior limbic keratoconjunctivitis
       (SLK) 37
Superior oblique muscle 91, 122
Superior rectus muscle 50, 52-53
Superior tarsus muscle 50
Surgery (eye) 104, 117-126, 156
Swelling *see* Edema
Sympathetic nervous system 27-28, 39
Symptoms 16, 18, 27-31, 33-35, 38,
       40-43, 45-47, 60
T2 Relaxation 95
T3 22, 146
T4 146-147

Taping eyes 61, 106-107, 155
Tarsorraphy 125
Tear duct plugs 108
Tear film 21, 33, 56-57
Tear supplements 106-108
Tearing 15, 27, 29, 31, 33, 36, 38-39,
       45, 47, 58, 60
Tears 49, 56
Tendons (eye) 50, 57, 119
Tensilon test 91, 99
Thyroglobulin 72
Thyroglobulin antibodies 20
Thyroid antibodies 20-21, 29, 63-65,
       83-84, 131
Thyroid cancer 20, 25
Thyroid disease 11, 20, 83
Thyroid eye disease 19-10, 37-38
Thyroid frown 27, 38
Thyroid hormone 21, 23, 28, 37-38, 30,
       48, 59, 67, 69, 75, 78-79, 85, 101,
       131, 142
Thyroid Manager 47
Thyroid ophthalmopathy 18
Thyroid peroxidase (TPO) antibodies
       20, 65, 83, 86
Thyroid-stimulating hormone (TSH) 18,
       22, 85
Thyroid stimulating immunoglobulins
       (TSI) 20, 44, 65, 67, 86, 90, 142,
       145, 149, 151
Thyroid storm 141
Thyroid surgery 113
Thyroiditis 20, 25
Thyrotoxicosis 25-26, 48
Thyrotropin *see* Thyroid-stimulating
       hormone (TSH)
Timeframe 20, 30, 40, 44-45, 105
Tonometry 89
Torsional strabismus 25
Torticollis 90
Tranquilizers 57, 81, 108
Treatment 13, 43-45, 48, 101-127
TSH *see* Thyroid-stimulating hormone
TSH receptor antibodies 20-21, 25,
       63-65, 67, 69-73, 77, 79, 83-86
TSH receptor protein 64-65, 69-70, 72

Tumor necrosis factor (TNF) 66
Tumors 32, 57, 96-97
Ulceration 39, 43, 45, 60
Ultrasonography 19, 84, 95, 97
Ultraviolet light 54
Unilateral proptosis 40, 97
Unilateral symptoms 31, 40
Upper eyelid 33, 38, 49, 99, 127
Upward gaze 35, 39, 46, 59, 61
Vigouroux's sign 33
Vision 50-51, 63
Visual acuity 29, 46-47, 86-87
Visual axis 34, 52
Visual evoked potentials 87
Visual field defects 29, 45
Visual field testing 87

Visual impairment 38, 43, 47
Visual loss 18, 38-39, 45-46, 55, 60, 121
Vitamin A 98
Vitamin B 135-136
Vitamin C 81
Vitreous humor 17, 32, 51, 54
Von Graefe's sign 32
Water 13
Watering see Tearing
Werner, Sidney 46
White blood cells 16-18, 29, 59, 63-65, 68-69
Women 77
Zinn's annulus 52
Zonule fibers 51

ISBN 141200911-1